ADVANCE PRAISE

We all know how to be healthy. This book is so different than any health book I have read. It forces you out of your own BS and kicks your butt into living that healthy lifestyle that you already know you should be living!

-Brittany Wisniewski, Best-selling author of
Keeping Well - an anti-cancer guide to remain in remission

Very interesting and informing book on how to get happy and healthy in return. Easy to read and follow. Great job, thank you for writing about something that is useful for everyone who chooses to take the time to do it.

-Blanch Beckes, Retired school bus driver

This book offers a unique perspective in that the author not only has expertise in the area of fitness, but she is also a Certified Transformational Coach. The result is that you gain personal insight which enables you to get to the root cause of the issue; then she shows you how to create a pro-active plan rather than just treat symptoms. The bonus is Ms. Graniel's humorous, delightful and refreshing view-point on the topic.

-Libby Adams, Ph.D., Founder of the International Academy of Self-Knowledge

GET HAPPIER & HEALTHIER NOW

GET HAPPIER & HEALTHIER NOW

7-Steps to Improved Health and a Body You Can Love

ELL GRANIEL

MOUNT TABOR MEDIA

NEW YORK

LONDON • NASHVILLE • MELBOURNE • VANCOUVER

Get Happier & Healthier Now

7-Steps to Improved Health and a Body You Can Love

© 2021 Ell Graniel

Published in New York, New York, by Mount Tabor Media, a branded imprint of Morgan James Publishing in partnership with Difference Press. Morgan James is a trademark of Morgan James, LLC. www.MorganJamesPublishing.com

ISBN 9781642799316 paperback
ISBN 9781642799323 eBook
Library of Congress Control Number: 2019955318

Cover & Interior Design by:
Christopher Kirk
www.GFSstudio.com

Editor:
Emily Tuttle

Book Coaching:
The Author Incubator

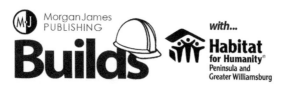

Morgan James is a proud partner of Habitat for Humanity Peninsula and Greater Williamsburg. Partners in building since 2006.

Get involved today! Visit
MorganJamesPublishing.com/giving-back

*This book is dedicated to all you brave souls
who have had enough, are ready
to reclaim your power, and take action
ripple, ripple, flutter, flutter.
I support and salute you!*

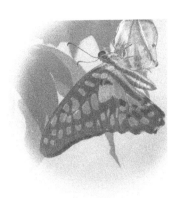

TABLE OF CONTENTS

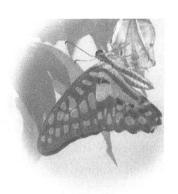

FOREWORD

Hello to all the readers of this book! My name is Dr. Rachel Reinhart Taylor, best-selling author of *Medication Detox* and board-certified Family Medicine physician. Early in my career I realized that although there is a time and place for Western Medicine, we have stopped relying on trusting our own intuition and bodies. In some cases, medications can end up being more harmful and a band-aid to cover symptoms instead of a real cure. I know Ell Graniel personally and have found that she has a passion for helping people honor and respect their own bodies and emotions to create REAL healing.

Ell has been a transformational coach for many years. Through her own personal and experience with her clients she has become an innovative mind in weight loss. She shows in this book how no matter what you do, there will not be a sustained change on the *outside* until there is a sustained change on the *inside*. She also details just how to do that with loving compassion. Ell gives great assignments that put the theoretical information into practical use. She does it all with such great humor too. Her ability to have fun while making changes assist people in finally getting the help they need and stop beating themselves up. Her approach is both refreshing and empowering for all of her readers. All too much we blame our "flaws" on ourselves and beat ourselves up. In my practice I see patients try every option including extreme diets, exercise, personal trainers, medications and surgery who find themselves angry at themselves when something hasn't worked. Ell has taken the pain out of getting both happy AND healthy through a reasonable program of weight loss that changes the whole human-mentally, emotionally, and spiritually.

I wrote this forward because I feel that people who have lost hope will have found some here through Ell Graniel's work. She is an inspiration for anybody who would like a permanent change in both the inside and outside. Even if you feel there is no hope and you think you've tried everything, don't give up. Ell will guide you through the steps it takes to come out victorious and show yourself you have what it takes.

Rachel Reinhart Taylor M.D.
Drreinharttaylor.com
Author: *Medication Detox: How to Live our Best Health, Simplified*

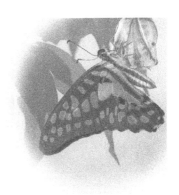

Introduction:

How You Got Here

Your past validation journeys

Welcome!
You're here now, with this book in your hands, because you have more self-motivation and tenacity than you give yourself credit for. You don't admit it openly because you are either too proud or have given up, but you truly desire to be in better health again, and finally off any medications for your overweight conditions.

In many cases, it's very challenging to even *talk* about your conditions and concerns for your long-term health and wellness. In one camp, you have family who say,

"It's hereditary, and there's not much you can do about it, because it's not your fault." And in the other camp, you have the ones who are neither happy or healthy, but want you to know it's okay and not your fault – because misery loves company.

However, you know you want to change because it hasn't always been this way. You want to be healthy again. You want to live a long and happy life, see the kids married, know the grandkids, see the world, and die peacefully in your sleep – with both legs and not dependent on a wheelchair, oxygen tank, or supervision. This is not too much to hope for. The only thing that has been holding you back from a healthy body is the major misconception that there are *magic numbers* and pills, which hold the keys to better, lasting health.

You're familiar with the nice, little statistical bell curve that considers your age, gender, and height to determine the healthy weight range for your body. In other words, the *magic number* that will haunt you for as long as you give it the power. A more accurate magic number would factor in muscle to bone ratios, whether you have an active or sedentary lifestyle, or even where you live geographically and the seasons.

Finally, it's worth mentioning that the way we have been taught to achieve that *magic number* is more fairytale than fact. But wait! I see some of you with your hand shooting up to remind me about the BMI (Body Mass Index). Sorry to disappoint, but that's another magic number based on the same overly general guidelines. Yes, it does ask you to input whether you are "normal or athletic," (WTH are those guidelines?) yet, it's calculations are still influenced by many factors, such as the time of day, how hydrated you are, or even whether you are sitting or standing.

Think of it like this... you know how when you ask Google for directions to say, an event in town? At some point, after it's done bossing you around, and sometimes not even talking to you for a bit, you hear, "You have arrived at your destination." The magic numbers are like that, in the sense that they are just "guides" which don't take into consideration important facts like: you need to park around the corner, then you need to find an elevator from the garage to the lobby, then yet another elevator to the floor of your event before you have truly, *arrived*. Basically, the **true** end result is missing a lot of facts.

So, let's get started by profiling the three most common scenarios people may go through, which often end at the same result... unhappy and unhealthy.

The most common scenario: I was a skinny kid who didn't know how amazing I was. In fact, I was so scrawny, I remember being made fun of.

This begins with you either being athletic, or very focused on a talent, like music or art. You were a kid with a great metabolism so you never thought about what you ate or imagined that you would ever be unhappy and overweight, even if you had family members who were. Then puberty came, and if you were in sports you stayed fit. But if you were into the arts, the weight began to show.

We'll address the arts later, but for now let's focus on the athlete. In junior high and high-school you most likely stayed fit – but then came your first "hit". Because you had muscle, you weighed more than the *magic number*, which was a red flag and your physician or parents became concerned. This is when the ride on the roller coaster of unhealthy weight gain and loss began. Some sports needed you to gain weight, like football, while others like wrestling and cheerleading required you to lose weight. So, the focus went off being happy and healthy, and onto what the scale said. And, I'll wager my favorite gold pumps that to this day, you are still a slave to the scale.

Sadly, either way, focus on weight gain or loss in the formative physical years of your life messed with your natural path to health. Those "diets" of the past have led you to believe that if you could only eat better and exercise again, you'd be healthy,

However, that's a fallacy, and antiquated thought that needs to be rectified before you can get back to healthy again. *Not* back to the body of your fit youth, but to the body of radiant health you can have now. That is to say, even when you get fit again, your body will be *very* different from the one you had in the past. Especially in its dimensions.

Next, we have the same beginning, but puberty was different if you were into the arts. You were a scrawny kid who maybe played sports and was active, then settled into a less physical life for the love of your artistic talent. Soon enough, you began to get "soft" and life went one of two ways. Either your overweight parents were so proud of your talent that they never talked about your weight – except once a year at the physical, where your doctor brought it up by pulling out the "magic number" bell curve that was defined by your age, height, and gender. Then, you and your parents were told to consider going on a "diet."

Or, your parents became "worried" about your weight and social status at school, so they put you on a "diet" on their own. Either way, the emphasis was on the "magic number" and that forced the distraction from happy, healthy living, to counting calories and not feeling "attractive" enough.

Now, when I mention that this next scenario was less common, I'm referring to the 1950s and 1960s. However, Gen X parents have reversed it to chubby being more common than skinny. Sadly, it has been predicted that children born to Gen X or even Millennials may be the first generation to die *before* their parents - due to obesity related diseases.

Time to profile the chubby kid. This is actually the toughest scenario, because either your parents were obese, in which case "chubby" was just fine, which allowed you to never explore healthy living, or they became worried about you becoming like them and thus began the feeling of "there's something wrong with me."

By the way - "Obese" means have eaten until fat.

Since the pattern of the "magic number" had been first set in your psyche, you became aware that you were either too heavy or too skinny as you moved through your college or post high school years.

Ever heard the term, "Freshman Fifteen"? In other countries, it's called the "Fresher Spread, First Year Fatties" or "Fresher Five." In my day, it was actually only ten pounds. Anyway, whether you were in college or not, it became acceptable to gain weight. The trouble with this forgiveness was that it assumed, once you got into a "normal" schedule, you'd be able to lose the weight. And yet, that magic number still eluded and haunted you, until one day you decided to give up and give in to the fact that you'd just never be that fit again - and that's okay. Besides, most of your friends were right there with you.

During this time, it most likely looked like this, "Yay! I'm out of the house and I can eat whatever I want." If instead, we had a solid conversation with ourselves about what we really wanted/desired, things could be different. But hey, who talks to themselves about that kind of stuff when they're nineteen – right? But if you had, it would have been easier than you thought, because you were out of the house and away from the influence of family and old habits. You could have chosen a different path for yourself

- one of happy *and* healthy. But you just honestly had no idea that was an option.

Okay, so what if you didn't go away and still lived at home while either working or going to the local college? Guess what, you could still gain the weight and people would look the other way because saying something to you would have meant having to live up to their own advice. Ugh! Again, either way, at a time when you could have been planning a happy, healthy lifestyle, you didn't have to, because basically no one cared enough – yet.

Now of course, there are lots of details I'm not covering. And, you could be a blend of the prior scenarios or possibly none of them. The point is, in these scenarios, this was your first opportunity to set up a lifestyle that included everything you love - all the things you enjoy, paired with the knowledge that *moderation* is all-powerful. Too much of most anything has unhealthy consequences. Not that you need to think in terms of 100% balance, but more along the lines of adding more of what you *know* is good for you (like walking), and *moderating* what you love – like pizza, beer, and TV – that may not be not so healthy. And you *know* that!

As we move on, it's important to understand that we're looking to live a life rich in things that make you laugh and smile, feel loved and appreciated, and overall happy. It's time to kick to the curb feelings of inadequacy, dependence on the acceptance of others, and above all else – that "magic number."

This part of the book is intended to assist you in taking back your power so you can get happy and healthy again – by choice, with passion and commitment. Are you ready to take back your power, stand up and claim it?! If "yes" then stand up and say, "The time is NOW to reclaim my health!"

At this point it may be hard to believe, but you can be happy, healthy, and still overweight.

When you understand and embrace this new way of thinking - that thin does not necessarily imply healthy - you'll be able to make changes to support a healthy lifestyle. This does not in any way mean diets and exercise! What it means is, your thoughts about your body, including body image and societal influences must get healthier before you can. Stay with me here...

Before we get into the actual seven-step process, let's address three primary reasons why you are still in the situation you're in:

1) your guilt
2) lack of awareness
3) wardrobe allowance

Ideally, your awareness of this knowledge can motivate you to begin taking back control.

First, your feelings of guilt. It's easy to understand how you could be feeling guilty for not trying harder, embarrassed to let others know what meds you're on, or hopeless about how you'll ever turn this around, because you sure you have tried. I believe you.

However, the truth is simple, as corny as it sounds... Today is a gift and the first day of the rest of your life. So, trust me when I tell you, you can have a healthy body as soon as you stop trying to just lose weight.

Second, your lack of awareness. You have *accepted* this situation you are living. Change that by harnessing the power of your awareness and writing down all the reasons why you are overweight and unhappy – without judgement or feelings of resentment – just the facts, as you see them. This will help you make a plan for what you *do want*, instead of what you *don't*.

Third, your wardrobe. You've allowed a one-size-fits-all closet! Stop the yo-yo of weight gain and loss by no longer allowing it in your wardrobe. Do this immediately. Go ahead and even stop reading to do it – it's very liberating. As Marie Kondo from "Tidying Up" suggests, put *every* single piece of clothing you own on your bed – including what's in your drawers, under your bed, and any other storage space. Then, besides just asking if they "spark joy" in you, ask yourself, "Does this fit me right now?" Anything that is either your skinny motivation or chubby allowance must go – no exception!

Your closet will now be suited for the body you are in at this time. You may no longer be depressed by clothes you are too fat for or allow yourself to gain weight because you know you still have things to wear (aka: fat clothes). When you open your closet, you should know everything in there fits and tells your story, personality, and brand. If things start getting tight, that's the cue telling you that you've been allowing outside influences to affect your health and body, so you can quickly address the source and get back to healthy, happy living. Everything in your closet will represent where you are today. Always.

I'm not a fan of using pain as a motivator but having to buy bigger clothes because nothing in your closet fits anymore will ideally be motivation enough for you to get back to actions where you feel most happy and healthy.

"Please, just the facts ma'am."

Remember the D.A.R.E. campaign? Well let's do that for ourselves but change the acronym to Drug, Awareness, Resistance, Education.

I have two questions. How do you feel on your meds? Are you happy with the fact that perhaps the side effects are worth it, because they are allowing you to become healthy again? Okay, one more question. Do you believe meds are your only or best option? Forgive me, one more. Is your physician overweight or have they offered any advice on possible healthy alternatives? Curious minds want to know.

This would also be a good time to mention the side effects they don't have to list on your meds, because they are just symptoms of being overweight...snoring, sleeplessness, sciatica pain, plantar fasciitis, knee and lower back pain, depression, hypertension, diabetes, and lethargy (to name a few). Note: most of these have a med to solve the "problem," but only as long as you keep taking them. Hmmm…now it's starting to look exponentially like meds, side effects, meds, side effects.

If you're ready to believe there's hope and a different way to approach your thoughts and actions about your overall long-term wellness, then let's jump into to the next exciting chapter about "chaos theory" and how you let it keep you fat. Remember, you're now stepping off the "ignorance is bliss" train, and onto the *awareness* train for the remainder of, not only this book, but the rest of your life. You will always know what you've read. It's only through awareness, followed by correct action, that lasting change can happen.

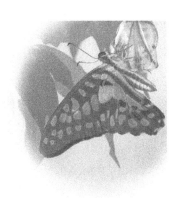

Chapter 1:

CHAOS AND THE BUTTERFLY EFFECT

Just When You Think Things Can't Get Any Worse...

As human beings, it's important to understand how fragile our lives are in terms of actual comfort and stability. When you truly believe the fact that every day is a miracle, and you live it on purpose, the happier and healthier you will be. That's not to say that "bad" things don't ever happen to "good" people. It simply means, when we spend time outside of gratitude and the moment, it's more likely we will energetically draw in chaos. And when we live our lives with intention and purpose, we can create a ripple or butterfly effect that touches the world.

What does this have to do with your weight? It means that you have the power and control to achieve all you desire, for better or worse, and especially when it comes to your health, weight, and happiness.

When we need reasons or excuses, we draw drama and chaos into our lives, so we can overeat, make poor food choices, and not get out to move our bodies in an enjoyable way. Chaos, however, is also a great tool for lasting change when you embrace it – since you invited it – and search for its true meaning. When you "get it," it passes and you are now living a life that is happier and healthier, by your own creation. If you choose to wallow in the suffering, you stay on the same path and no matter how hard you "try," the weight will always come back – usually with a vengeance.

There are several definitions of chaos, from scientific to linguistic. However, the one I enjoy most is the one defined by Michael Crichton in his novel *Jurassic Park*. Each chapter moves through the theory of chaos until you hit the best part, "When you think things can't get any worse, they do!" The good news is, you are still actually in control of it, when you embrace it and know you will get through it sooner when you seek the message it brings. Sometimes, you'll really have to dig deep. And sometimes, they say, the best way to get out of the hole you've dug yourself in, is to simply put down the shovel. That's the beauty of chaos. It's up to you to decide how to ride it out.

It may sound crazy, but when stuff starts to hit the fan for me, I sometimes go outside (in bare feet) onto the grass, throw my hands to the heavens and say "*Bring it. I'm ready, willing, and able.*" Then I unleash a big, deep, heartfelt belly laugh, which sometimes brings me to tears. After that, things seem to get better. If that's not an option or something I feel like doing, then a big snotty nose, curled up in fetal pose, hot shower cry also works. Uh, until the water runs cold.

Now, let's look at a few less scary lifestyle choices you're making that need attention...

If you haven't seen the movie *Groundhog Day*, watch it (or watch it again). This is a fun way to help you see how you are doing the same thing every day and are not happy or healthy. The main lesson is not actually to do things differently, like fad diets, but to get to what makes you happy – then things will shift. So, stop gaining and losing those ten plus groundhog pounds and look at what's making you so unhappy that you stay stuck in those "bad" choices.

Write down the baby steps you are ready to take in making change. Pick some easy things you can do like quit diet soda (because it's also actually killing you) and once those become "natural" to you, step up to a bigger challenge. Before you know it, you'll no longer be eating fast food, drinking diet soda, and maybe you'll even be enjoying a walk after dinner – and, actually looking forward to it. And, so will the dog!

Next, you need to look at all the people you surround yourself with that support you in your unhealthy, med-induced lifestyle. It's human nature to not like change and avoid it at all costs. However, you eased into the way you live now, and you can ease out of it. Sadly, when you start getting healthy and taking the action steps, loved ones will notice and may start to support you - with their words. But, their actions will not. Because, when you change, and start acting healthy, they will have to also. And they sure don't want that! As the saying goes, "Misery loves company." So, this is your chance to create a beautiful butterfly effect. Do it for yourself and no single other reason. The butterfly effect is a concept where small causes (actions) can have large effects. A great example is how a walk after dinner can lead to improved circulation, mental clarity, and positive attitude.

Here are a few stories I believe you will find relatable or encouraging:

First, *mine*! I was that scrawny kid who was made fun of in elementary school. When my sister (who was also scrawny) and I would trick or treat for UNICEF, people would jokingly say, "Keep the money for yourself." Then, I got into softball and started to get some muscles. I continued through high school, playing sports with a killer metabolism. I even began lifting weights and truly loved my body – and it loved me! That's not to say I was confident; I was just healthy, and I knew it. Then, I left for college, and without playing sports (because I wasn't *that* good) I gained nearly twenty pounds! I was for sure a "Freshman Fatty".

Basically, if you're not moving your body every day, you need to make even better food choices and introduce yourself to moderation, aka: portion control. So, when I came home for summer break and didn't want to go to the lake because I no longer loved my body, it began to not love me back and I started to suffer from a series of "ailments." I remember spending that summer feeling like an outsider in my own hometown because my body no longer represented who I felt I was, a sexy, independent woman. It didn't help that my boyfriend dumped me less than a week after I got home for a fitter, sexier gal.

I worked a full and part-time job that helped pay my bills when I went back to college. I used them as excuses for not socializing. I felt depressed and preferred to stay home. And since my dad was "away," there was no one to question me. When I did go out, I put on a happy face and pretended everything was hunky dory. Especially for my mom, who had me over for dinner every evening in the two-hour break between my jobs. This was also the first time I started having digestive issues, aches in my body first thing in the morning, and grumpiness.

Shortly thereafter, I found the wonderful world of self-help and began to love my body again. With the guru wisdom of Zig Ziglar, Dr. Wayne Dyer, and the Earl Nightingale motivational club, getting back to my ideal size eight was actually easy because my passion for being happy and healthy was back. After that, my weight ebbed and flowed with marriage, multiple careers, two kids, some chaos, divorce, and a quick bout with depression while writing my first book. As I got older, I bumped up to a comfortable size twelve and was told the lie we like to believe, "It's okay. As you age, your metabolism slows."

Side Note: Your metabolism does not slow. It adapts. If you slow for long periods of time, after storing fat, it slows to ensure your long-term survival. And, it is very apprehensive to pick up again. But it will.

Anyway, twenty years flew by and I met my second husband, who was a doting chef. Within one year, I gained nearly thirty-five pounds of what I called "happy fat". Here is the important part of this story...even though I was fifty pounds overweight – according to the magic number the doctors go by – I was healthy! My cholesterol, blood sugar, and blood pressure were all in the healthy range. However, I was snoring, got plantar fasciitis, sciatic pain, and my libido died. Want to hear the good part? My doctor did not tell me to lose weight to feel good again. Go ahead and guess what happened...yup, meds.

Funny thing is, when I asked my doctor (who was overweight) if my foot pain would go away if I just lost about twenty pounds, he said, "Not necessarily." *Wow*!

Okay, so ten years pass and then some more chaos with the sudden passing of hubby, and within one year, I lost thirty pounds. Not from depression but from not being fed delicious, high calorie food every day anymore. Lucky for me, my cooking has never been that wonderful so it's easy for me to stop eating when I'm full. Here's the kicker, when I got my blood work done, my numbers were still the same – healthy! How is it possible that I could be thirty pounds lighter and still have the same numbers? Okay fine, I'll tell you...it's because it is not about the numbers, it's about "quality of life." I was happy with my life then and now.

That brings us to today. I've been itching to write a follow up to my first self-published book back in 2006, *Chocolate Cake for the Thighs*. That first book was just plain fun. I've always loved writing, public speaking, and dancing (not professionally, more disco duck), which somehow led to a long-term career in the fitness world. Whenever I taught classes I would always end with a fitness tip that I made up, based on my then ten plus years of certifications and continuing education. If I forgot to give one, the ladies would always remind me, and some mentioned putting them into a book. Bam! The lightbulb went on and I began to write my tips down. After a few months of chronicling them, I realized I had one hundred and one, a great start on the title. I combined my decade of self-help and motivation with fitness and the book practically wrote itself.

This year I promised myself I'd get an agent and speak the message of happy and healthy (without diets and exercise) in greater detail to my audience, who is now nearly fourteen years older. I'm taking the message much more seriously, because now, lives are at stake.

This time I wanted the learning to stick and become a lifestyle that's realistic *and* enjoyable.

Since I preach "action burns way more calories than all talk," I found the perfect agent for my message. Shortly thereafter, she was being featured at the Palm Springs Documentary Film Festival, and I was extended a limited invitation to attend. It was an amazing confirmation that I was on the right path. Especially when I got my picture taken with her on the red carpet! It was surreal.

On the last evening of the event, I had dinner with friends and when returning to my hotel, I fractured my foot by not being mindful and missing a step down. It could have been worse. I could have fractured my hand and not been able to write! Or hit my head and forgot I was even writing a book. Now, I'm still in recovery for a couple more weeks and I can't teach my favorite fitness classes. Rather than change my diet, I've just allowed myself to keep on keeping on. And as I sit here typing, I weigh twelve pounds more than before my accident. Yup, twelve pounds in just eleven weeks, and I'm embracing it because I know with confidence, it's temporary. As soon as I can get back to my beloved group fitness gals, the fat will melt away. I choose to stay optimistic.

Now calm down, I know I said no exercise, yet here I am a fitness instructor. You may be thinking it must be easy for me to keep the weight off with all that exercise. Technically, I do not teach exercise classes, nor do I exercise (we'll elaborate on this later). I teach fitness classes and I enjoy moving my body every day. "Semantics" you might say. "Yes," however, choosing the best words that truly express your thoughts, feelings, and desires is crucial to your overall health and happiness. If you hang in here for just a bit longer, you'll learn how to do that for yourself easily. I'm laughing to myself right now thinking about how when I shed the twelve pounds I gained during my "learning experience," I'll still be fifteen pounds over that *magic number.* And yet very happy, healthy, and med-free.

Next up, Jim

Jim's weight has ebbed and flowed with the chaos that is life: divorce, being estranged from his kids, a soul-sucking job, and a few scattered injuries.

Jim was an artist, not an athlete, as a kid, who was always chubby. Since everyone else in his family was overweight, it didn't bother him until junior high when he noticed only the chubby girls liked him. But he didn't want the chubby girls to like him, he wanted Sheila! So, at the influential age of thirteen, he went on his first diet, messing with his developing metabolism. And guess what? He lost weight, but it didn't get him Sheila, so he went off the diet and gained back even more weight.

By the time high school came around, he was on two meds. He had a horrific experience when at band camp (yes, band camp) when his meds were found, and the kids started a rumor that he was on drugs. After several decades of roller coaster rides with weight loss, he came to me, thinking being thinner would make him happy. Jim then finally decided to forget about dieting and just concentrate on his music, and guess what? Yup, he lost ten pounds and got off both meds. He's actually still fifty pounds overweight, yet ten pounds lighter was the *real* magic number for him.

To this date (eighteen years later), Jim gains weight very easily and blames it on dieting at a young age. He jokes that he can gain weight just by looking at food. He's just about forty pounds overweight and feels great. He is happy, healthy, and med-free.

Linda

Linda never really had to think about her weight. She enjoyed fruits and vegetables, as well as pizza and pasta. She loved the outdoors and walking her dogs. Then, in her thirties, Linda got on the fast track at work as an investment portfolio manager. This brought long stressful hours at work and deadlines with profits on the line every day. Soon she was addicted to caffeine, eating at her desk, working weekends, and only walking the dogs once a day. Sometimes, she even had to hire a dog walker. As Linda began to gain weight, she developed an ulcer, and had to get on meds for hypertension and high cholesterol.

We met at one of my fitness classes, when she decided she didn't want to die young and alone. Together we uncovered that Linda's plan was to just start working out again with daily dog walks and yoga – great baby steps/butterfly effect. That led to wanting to become a yoga instructor and student of meditation. Soon the ulcer went away – even though she still drinks coffee – and she got off the meds. I credit her leap of faith as the true catalyst for her lasting success, which is over ten years now. Linda decided to quit her twenty-year career to become a yoga instructor and a start an outdoor activity business where she leads hiking and kayaking tours. Oh, and she'll celebrate her ten-year anniversary to her very outdoorsy hubby this year.

Mary

Mary's story is short. She came to me this year because she can't gain weight and is on meds for hypertension and diabetes. She has always been thin, sinewy, and fidgety. Because she can eat whatever she wants, she does - especially simple carbs. And, when life gets chaotic, she loses even more weight, to the point of becoming dangerously underweight! Please note that you can be thin and still be on the same meds as overweight, unhealthy people.

But now, Mary is healthy because she is choosing to lead by example for her three kids and show them what healthy eating looks like. Before, she ate her feelings. Today, she's learned how to recognize her "triggers" and deals with them right on the spot. Her weight ebbs and flows by ten pounds and she is happily off the meds.

I hope you are getting the idea of how it's possible to get happier and healthier, **and** that it's not the way you've been doing it.

In the next chapter, we'll layout the options for creating a happy, healthy life and body. Need help identifying your triggers? Stay tuned...

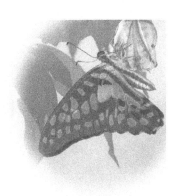

Chapter 2:

THE ROAD MAP

The How of Why It's Going to Be Different This Time

Many are familiar with Einstein's definition of insanity. So why then, did poor Phil in the movie *Groundhog Day* starring Bill Murray continue to suffer insanity, even though he did several things differently every day? Because, he did not know what outcome he truly wanted. Only when he surrendered to the chaos did he find what really made him happy and was released to live his life on purpose with direction and passion.

This chapter is all about what you're ready, willing, and able to surrender to so you can lose weight, and live a happy, healthy life.

First, as your benevolent leader, let me explain *how* to get the most out of this book. I recommend you get a highlighter and glide it along everything that calls to you on your first read through *before* you do the assignments. Maybe you can relate to it, want more of that, or just feel like it's worth noting. This way, you can breeze through the messages, knowing you can take more inspired action *after* you see the big picture.

If you instead choose to tackle the assignments as we go, statistics are, you'll get stuck there and never get back (a subconscious sabotage). In the words of my all-time famous motivational speaker, Zig Ziglar*, "You'll get baked in the squat." meaning you'll never rise to your fullest potential.

Also, wherever you see the *, it's marking a term in the "google section" of the reference page, where you can learn a bit more about these fascinating topics.

It is my passion that you will never again be a statistic. I prefer we be *outliers* or *mavericks*, in the terms of Malcolm Gladwell's books on statistics and success*. The highlight reading technique will also allow you to pick and choose what is "junk," meaning not relatable to you and your current circumstance, and what to tackle first, with confidence, passion, and joy. I've already tossed out a few assignments in the previous chapters, and if you've started them already, *super*, but stop! Just wait until you've finished the book, which won't take long, since it's not a novel. If you'll trust me on this, not only will you avoid being a "squat" statistic, but your overall success will come more naturally and last a lifetime – or as long as you want it.

I already told you my story about my fractured foot, so now I can expand on unrealistic timelines and expectations. When the doctor first looked at the x-ray, she said, "Well, at your age, you should expect at least twelve weeks for a full recovery." At my age! Humph, did she not know I was happy and healthy, my numbers were good – including bone density – and that her diagnosis was *way* off? I set my mind to eight weeks – a full four weeks early – for recovery. I would show them. I'm never a statistic... Um, never say never.

So, I set to work with upping my calcium, and doing everything the doc said (except take the three meds prescribed for pain, inflammation, and to help me sleep because those were not even issues for me). I had daily massages with my oils, Epsom salt foot soaks, and the full R.I.C.E. applications. When I meditated, I imagined beautiful hummingbirds dropping calcium into the little cracks of my bone and smoothing it over with their wings. I was going to be a medical miracle and show them! Well, guess what? As I rolled into week twelve of recovery, she was right. I'm going to be released back to teaching in about ten days – a full thirteen weeks later.

I'll bet you didn't think it was going to go like that – am I right? Me either. Looking back, I believe the reason why I became that statistic is simple; I was too focused on proving the stats wrong and not on just living my life with joy for where I was on this journey. I was often thinking about everything I was missing out on and was frustrated. In the words of Tad James, PhD, "There are no unrealistic goals, only unrealistic time frames."

If only, in hindsight, I had gone outside with my feet in the grass and my hands to the sky, embracing the chaos, and shouting "*Bring it! I'm ready willing and able!*" I'm positive things could have been different. I'm not saying I would have had the eight-week recovery (although that's possible), what I'm sharing with you as you travel though everything this process brings up for you, is to look it right in the eye, thank it for what you are about to learn or are learning, and become a front row student majoring in awareness.

I now know more about my patience, how to be alone, how to talk to all the voices in my head from a place of compassion, and that I actually wouldn't die if I couldn't teach my beloved classes for three months.

Embrace the chaos and say, "I brought this, I've got this!" and then get quiet and pay attention.

Okay, after your first highlighted run through, then it's time to go back and make your plan of baby steps (butterfly effect). Why you are here, in this body, was a series of baby steps. You didn't just wake up one day overweight, unhealthy, unhappy with your life and on meds. No, it was a series of choices that can now be *unchosen* because you are ready.

I'd like to throw in a potential deal-breaker here. Please be hyper-aware that once you take the lid off the proverbial trash can, it's going to stink for a while. Your ego, the poster child hater of change, is going to get loud and rowdy. It's up to you to stay large and in charge... and here's how.

1. Get a journal or just plain notebook that is *specifically* for this work – use it every day and do your best to have it nearby, always.

2. Create a space, like a dropbox file where you can keep everything. Put your journal notes there every day or use your phone and make voice notes and video clips to store there as well.

3. Make a good motivational playlist – edit it as you evolve and allow it to keep you on track (hint: I'm already creating one for you with every chapter) or you can use mine, if you have a Spotify account – email me for the link!

Side note: No sad, angry, or vindictive songs allowed. Even if they motivate you. This is an important shift in motivation you must bravely make.

Along the same vein, take a ninety-day hiatus from "dark" movies and the daily news as well. Avoid watching them and see how you blossom. If you need the news for work, listen to or read just what is relevant. Mark ninety days on your calendar because it's longer than you think, especially in this fast-paced life.

While working this process, notice what your ego is telling you. Write it down, and keep reminding it, "Thanks for sharing, but I make the decisions. Always have, always will."

Bonus: Begin to bring your awareness to your breath every time you feel you're about to make a "bad" choice. Stop for just a minute or two and take control. Breathe in deeply, feeling the air travel in from your nose or mouth and down your throat. Then, exhale slower and longer than normal while allowing your shoulders to relax and drop down and back away from your ears. Open your chest and allow more breath in and out. Keep this going for the remainder of the next few minutes while you close your eyes and gently massage your ears, temples, and jawline – spend extra time on your earlobes. If necessary, do this a hundred times a day as you learn how to take control back, away from your ego. Ignore my earlier advice about not doing the assignments yet and do this now.

Think about it... you can go without food and water for many days, but you can't go without breath for more than several minutes. Your breath is so vital to your life and you have so much control over how it happens! Start now by being more aware of how you breathe. Chances are, you're mostly getting in just enough survival breaths. When you begin to regularly breathe deeper and fuller, you switch to breaths that help you thrive. Your wellness is just one deep and meaningful breath away, so to speak. Also notice it's harder to hold tension in your jaw, shoulders, and gut when you are breathing big, both on the inhale and exhale. Take your time and play with how it feels, then find a rhythm that feels more natural for you.

But wait! Aren't we going to keep a food journal, get some healthy recipes, start counting our steps and calories, or join a gym? Nope, correct me if I'm wrong, but you've done most, if not all, of that – more than once – and here you are... so to copy the motivational anthem of Susan Powter, let's "Stop the insanity." Why waste time talking about how to eat better when you already know how? Our time will be spent on why you're *choosing* to *not* take the healthier actions. This is also a good place to remind you that I am not a doctor, dietitian, or nurse advising you to stop your meds, go on a diet, or start running (or any other crazy exercise).

This is all about eliminating the causes, not the symptoms (unlike meds – but I'm not saying "stop now"). It's time to finally stop trying to fix what's wrong and focus on what's right. And believe me or not, what's right is you! Here's the kicker, we're not even going to use goals, positive thinking, or affirmations because I'll wager my disco ball collection, you've already dabbled in that as well (without much lasting luck).

Remember, it's all about being healthy and that begins with your willingness to know you deserve it. The best road trips are the ones that allow for stops and detours along the way. The most stressful are the ones on time-tables with no margin for error, practically just inviting chaos as your navigator.

If you're still on board, it's time to dive into the seven-step process...

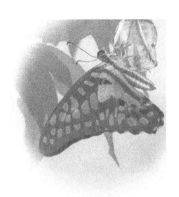

Chapter 3:

THE E.M.P.A.T.H.Y. WAY

Getting Back to the Body You Love, That Loves You Back

This is why every failure you've endured has brought you to the success you're about to achieve.

Before we dive into the seven-steps of E.M.P.A.T.H.Y. Way, let's review...

When you think about the things that have made you stronger and smarter, they usually involve chaos in some way – loss, epic failure, or basically most of the seven deadly sins (especially sloth and envy), as well as a few of the seven dwarfs. That's exactly how you know you're ready for success in the area of improved health and overall wellness. You've been there, done that. Now, it's time to channel all of that learning into one direction - getting healthy again.

Remember, you've already tried dieting, fitness fads, counting steps, calories, and positive thinking, just to eventually gain not only the weight back but even more because chronic dieting (and drinking diet soda) is associated with weight gain. One factor that contributes to this phenomenon is an increase in appetite hormones. In addition, calorie restriction and loss of muscle mass causes your body's metabolism to slow down, making it easier to regain weight once you start eating *normally* again. Also, when you lose weight quickly, especially without exercise, you not only lose fat, you lose muscle as well. And you may have to deal with other issues that contribute to weight gain, such as stress and a disrupted sleep pattern from your caloric chaos.

Therefore, this is not the solution (but you know that). Plus, as some of you learned, dieting in your prime, physical formative years has led your body to believe you are always one step away from famine – again – so it holds as much fat as possible to keep you "safe" even decades later. And some of you know that if you would just start being the athlete again, you'd get back in shape. But guess what? For some reason, you just can't bring yourself to do it again.

I stand firm on the fact that diets don't work. If they did, no one would be overweight. Yet, I hear people say, "Of course diets work. People lose weight on them all the time." To which I counter, "True, but rarely forever." You also lose weight when you get the flu, food poisoning, or take drugs like diuretics, amphetamines, or cocaine. But I hope you would not expose yourself to that just to lose weight. So, stop trying the diets and just eat better because you *know* how. Just saying. Baby steps please. It's very true that some of folks have "fad" dieted and kept the weight off, but they're not the ones reading this book.

Let's bust up the illusion of willpower and self-discipline, shall we? I see so many people hang their head in shame and pronounce, "If only I had willpower/self-discipline." You do! Begin adding to the list you're making, all the times you did stick with it - not the times you did not. Think of *all* those situations (not just the diet and exercise ones), then look at the circumstances that helped make them happen. I'll bet my baby beauty contest trophy (yes, I still have it) that you'll see a pattern of how "willpower" looks for you. Willpower is a talent. We all have it, it just looks different on everyone – kind of like jeans.

This is where your emotions come into play. Your body is designed for homeostasis. It seeks normalcy, complacency, and predictability. That's exactly why it's been so difficult to get back to the body you love. It has nothing to do with willpower. It's just been so long since you've been there that your body and mind have forgotten what it feels like and how happy it makes you.

The good news is, there is also something called muscle memory*. It's a super cool thing where, once your body has done something regularly, it's easier for it to bounce back to that state. This means that if you ever enjoyed some type of physical activity, no matter how many years ago, doing it again will bring a smile to your face, laughter in your heart, and after a few short days of DOMS (Delayed Onset Muscle Soreness), you'll be almost good as new. I say almost, because the body of your youth is still different from your adult body. Not better, just different. And different is good. Change is good because you're either green and growing or rotting.

I can't believe I'm saying this, but it's true...being overweight and unhappy/depressed isn't 100% your fault. That's hard for me to say because I'm a huge fan of personal responsibility and honesty. However, sometimes we just don't know. Like when we thought the world was flat, leeches pulled out illness, or that conditions just "run in the family."

As we move on, it's time to expose all the lies you've been led to believe so you can really let go of your guilt or hopelessness and get the body you love that loves you just as much! Then, you can create a reasonable plan of action that suits your current lifestyle. You're going to choose things you enjoy and make them a permanent part of how you live your life.

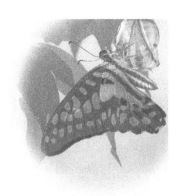

Chapter 4:

E – EMBRACING YOUR FAILURE

And the dreaded "E" word

You know how when something embarrassing happened to you, as you retold the story, people just cracked up laughing, including you? That's the idea behind this chapter.

Remember when you thought it was a good idea to wear legwarmers as part of your wardrobe? Or how you used to drink cheap wine? This chapter is like that. You will recall all the things you did, because you either didn't know any better or were just following the trends. Then, you'll take the best part of those experiences and turn them into something wonderful that supports you and gives you more confidence going forward.

Food for thought: Did you know the word diet means, the *way* you eat. *How* you eat is your diet. It doesn't mean eating less, restrictive or weird. There's those semantics again. Why eat plain toast, half a grapefruit, and black coffee if you don't *enjoy* it? I'm lucky, I truly enjoy black coffee (um, but only if it's my special blend from Mexico). Get this simple equation in your head. Make it a mantra even. Happy = Healthy

True story: When the South Beach diet was in its heyday, hubby and I decided to give it a try. I only agreed because I read the book and compared to all the other diets out there; it made sense. It was the first I'd seen that delved into clean eating.

Since I was the meal planner, prepper, and preparer at the time, it was clear that the whole family would be eating this way. Boy oh boy, you should have heard the lectures I got about putting my "scrawny" kids on a diet. And of course, people only knew we were "dieting" because the kids hated the South Beach (SB) desserts and told everyone they were forced to be on a diet. Anyway, the thing you need to know is, hubby and I both lost weight (only to gain it back later), but the kids – ages seven and twelve - did not lose a pound! Why? Because it was really about eliminating soda, refined sugar, and processed meats. To this day, over nineteen years later, I still don't drink soda because that "diet" helped eliminate it from my palate. And there are a few other good things I still eat which I learned in that process. However, I would never do it again. I learned what I needed to learn.

Side note: Drinking diet soda to lose weight is like trying to look healthier by tanning without sunscreen. It's downright dangerous and very unhealthy, so stop it! If you must have diet soda in the house, use it solely for cleaning rings from the toilet. You've seen that YouTube video, haven't you?

Begin embracing your failures! Find the lessons and the good within them to keep with you. Let the rest go as something you learned and will never do again, like the first time you touched something hot on the stove. But not like the first time you burnt the roof of your mouth on hot pizza. That's still a thing. I'm not trying to be contradictory here. I'm doing my best to help you see how it's all a journey with lots of life choices that can be determined by you – not your ego. My good friend Julie, will only eat pizza with a knife and fork because she claims it's the only way to never have a roof of the mouth blister ever again. She's my perfect example of an outlier and someone who figured out how to get a different outcome through a tested action. You could also just never eat pizza again, or just accept your consequences and eat the pizza even though you know it's hot - because this time you'll chew with your mouth open. See what I mean?

Embrace your failures and then either accept their lessons or keep getting burned. You have the power; no one forces you to eat hot pizza that is sure to burn the roof of your mouth because everyone knows it's rude to chew with your mouth open, right?

Next on the chopping block of lies you've been brainwashed into believing – and has kept you overweight - is the concept of calories. Just like the word "diet," most people don't know the actual definition of *calorie* is a unit of energy. What's so cool about this, is in other countries where obesity is not so much an issue, their food labels don't even say calories – instead, they say *energy*. So, when you read the label, you understand how much energy or fuel your body is getting. I never knew this until I visited my youngest in New Zealand. It was such an eye opener.

Instead, we have misconceptions like "energy drinks." But it gets even worse because...

Since we're on the subject of food label lies, let's get real about what they're (not) telling you. The first thing you see because it's usually bold, is "nutrition facts", which is already a joke because they are based on a 2,000-calorie-a-day diet. Therefore, the label should say "nutrition generalities" since for millions of people, this is already an inaccurate account of what they're really getting or needing (kind of like that magic weight number from the doctor's chart). The serving size is also a joke that comedians poke fun of regularly. The manufacturer can set the serving size to whatever they want to make the "facts" look more appealing.

I'm not picking on the Girl Scouts here because they do not make the serving size, but my favorite cookie is only two per serving! What? For me, portion control is four cookies. And comedian Brian Regan claims his portion is a sleeve. Then, how about Ben and Jerry's? Ever looked? Interesting how we rarely look at some food labels, or even worse, we read them while we're eating it – alas, but I digress. A pint of their ice cream is listed as one-half cup or four servings per pint. Have you ever shared a pint of ice cream with three other people? Not if you're still friends, I'll bet. So, basically now you know those "nutrition facts" are very loosey- goosey.

Lastly, let's put the *ingredients* on food labels under the microscope – and sometimes you literally have to, because the font is so teeny tiny or, they're on the seam, or where you tear it open. The one good thing I can say about this part (because I like finding the good) is that they must list the ingredients in order of the amount used in the product vs alphabetically. That's how you can see how little fruit is in your juice, for example.

But what I find entertaining is when they want you to know what the ingredient is, it looks like this: "Natamycin (a natural mold inhibitor)" or "TBHQ (to preserve fresh-ness)." But when they don't want you to *know*, it looks like this: "Cellulose," when it should look like this, "Cellulose (sawdust)." By the way, that's often what they use to keep shredded cheese from sticking to itself.

Are you aware you could grate your own cheese and toss it with just a slight dust of cornstarch for the same, much healthier effect? Here's a fun task. Give a list of the things on your food labels that you have no idea what they are to your kids and have them Google it for you. Now that you're all educated, shopping will be so much more fun!

One last giggle about nutrition facts. I love to laugh, so I appreciate it when the package of Red-Vines says, "Fat Free" or the lunchmeat says, "Gluten Free." That's such a good one.

If you'd like to use your phone for an agent of good, download one of the many amazing and educational apps that allow you to know exactly what you're eating, just by scanning the barcode! For example, you can be informed that Sodium Nitrate is also used in smoke bombs and pyrotechnics...cool.

Let's move on to the nutritional education we received growing up, which shapes our perception of "healthy" eating. Back in my day, when obesity was not an epidemic yet, we had the four part "square". You were encouraged to eat a meal consisting of dairy, meat, grains, and fruit/veggies, and to have three square meals a day to stay healthy. The concept was simple, just eat healthy because you *know* what healthy is and is not. Duh. Then after much lobbying, in the eighties the "Food Guide Pyramid" gained popularity. I don't have time to get into all the reasons why this is a horrible representation of healthy eating, but just check out the evolution of it*. Finally, in 2005, they improved the concept by switching the visual from horizontal blocks to vertical wedges.

Time to undo the magic, shall we? Let's move on to numbers and the ridiculousness of weight charts, BMI, and the daily sixty ounces of water mandate. I'm pretty sure you know this stuff, so I'll be brief because it's important and worth revisiting.

The weight chart the doctor uses includes factors such as age, height, and gender, which have nothing to do with lifestyle. Therefore, it is terribly inaccurate and just another misconception you've been led to believe. A perfect example of this is a side-by-side comparison of two of my clients. They are both five foot six, female, and about the same age and weight, but one wears a size ten and the other a size fourteen, even though their weight is only five pounds apart. As a rule of thumb for women, every ten pounds means the next size up. So, in "reality" the size fourteen gal should be twenty pounds heavier. Get my point?

I'm going to implore you to stop using the scale as a measurement of your health. It's like texting...so much gets lost in translation. Instead, use the more esoteric system of how you "feel" mentally, physically, emotionally, *and* especially in your clothes. It's a simple concept. When your clothes start getting tight, it's time to evaluate your life. A happy "fatty" can be med free and live a longer healthy life than a miserable skinny person.

Can I give you a new word? Are you ready? Let's all strive to become a "*Fittie.*" A *Fittie,* is someone who is happy and healthy – not a slave to the scale, diets, or step counting. Oh, and what you may not know, is that Body

Mass Index (BMI) is also a general number that does not take lifestyle into account. If you really, really, need to know your body fat percentage (even though I told you to stop looking at the numbers), the most accurate is the hydrostatic dunking process*. Plus, it's not that expensive. But hey, sometimes ignorance is bliss.

This brings us to the final and most critical reason why you're overweight and unhappy...The dreaded E word. Like how in the *Harry Potter* books there was the name you could not say out loud, I'd like you to make "exercise" that word for you. Here's why exercise has failed you. You've most likely been led to believe that it includes some sort of heart-pounding, sweaty activity and none of them call to you. You look at all the "fit" people running in the gym or on infomercials and feel hopeless because you've tried it and failed miserably. Or maybe you even lost a quick ten pounds and then quit because you hated it, then twelve pounds later you're beating yourself up – again.

Side note: Beating yourself up does not burn calories. Even though it may sound like exercise.

Discipline and exercise, ugh! Two of the least passionate words I know. Disagree? (It's really a military thing). How does this statement make you *feel*? "I really need to exercise some self-discipline in that area of my life." Is it motivational or not so much? More like beating yourself up again?

I'm about to make a few enemies here, but I'm not a fan of the 10,000 steps a day campaign. Actually, for lots of folks, it does more harm than good. Stay with me – here's why...First, have you ever tried it? It's super hard! Therefore, you feel like a failure and eat something to comfort your feelings. Or, you hit your steps, yay, so you eat something you "deserve" as a reward. Once the novelty wears off, unless you have an accountability partner to walk with, most likely, you will no longer be counting and if you did lose weight, it will come back. If counting steps is the best thing that ever happened to you, cheers! Just never call it exercise, or your ego might try and talk you out of it. Call it what it is, walking/stepping/running/jogging. Window shopping knocks out lots of steps! The one good thing that came out of the 10,000 daily challenge is that people finally started parking farther away in parking lots and walked to help get their steps in instead of sharking around wasting time, gas, and making pollution with their car.

How about you say to yourself every day, "Today I'm going to do something that moves me!" And then do it. If running/jogging/walking were the only ways to exercise and stay fit, I'd be dead already, because I despise all three. Running hurts and I find it boring. I hit what runners call "the wall" by the third mailbox. As a matter of fact, I seriously joke that if you ever see me running, you better start too, because something really bad is coming down the street. Jogging just emphasizes how much parts of me jiggle when I do it – ick. And, walking doesn't *move* me. It's just something you do because you are blessed enough to be able to do it. Stop thinking of the E word and start thinking about what *moves* you. Remember, you burn calories even while you're sleeping so stop thinking about exercise as a means to burning calories and start doing things you enjoy. Wait! I'm not saying sleep more. Although it is better for you than watching TV - to a point.

Over time you can take it up a notch, like going from walking the dogs to jogging, then running with them. Or from gardening and yard work, to landscaping. You get the idea. There are thousands of ways to move – start today. No more buts/excuses. Basically, get off your butt and do something. Get out of the house and ideally into nature. But if that's not an option, put on a killer playlist and get some housework done dance-style, or just plain dance around the house like Kevin Bacon and Chris Penn at the school in the movie *Footloose*. No more *exercise* for you!

From now on, you're literally a mover and a shaker! And if you can't break free of your mortal enemy, the TV, then get up and move during the commercials. No commercials? Then pick a character or talking head and get moving every time they are speaking. Just getting up and down for this alone will be an amazing start.

Like I said, if the 10,000 steps are working for you then keep on keeping on, because when you enjoy it then it's not the E word.

I'd be remiss if I didn't put in a word here against the media...You know those magazine ads are so touched up the models don't even have veins in their eyes – so creepy.

Then there's what the media decides we need to know... creepy, sad, depressing, dramatic, and mind-numbing.

Enough said, let's review.

Now you understand how your epic failures were a product of lies and misconceptions. And now you know why and how things are going to change – forever.

I'm so excited we've come to the time where you'll make a real plan for your life that suits who you are as a person, including your dreams and passions. This is now possible for you because you have learned how your past "mistakes" were just leading to this point so you can make decisions with confidence because you've "been there, done that." Are you ready to put the mental to the pedal?

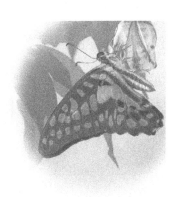

Chapter 5:

M – Making Decisions about What's Possible

It's Time to Get R.E.A.L. about Your Plan of Action

R.E.A.L. is another acronym for **Really Energized About Life**, but we'll get back to that later. I know you're thinking, "Come on, can you put an acronym in your acronyms?" Yup!

In my ongoing research into neuroscience and how the brain processes information, I fell in love with the simple application of association. Basically, it's easy to remember something when you can relate to it. My top three for long term retention are

1) acronyms
2) music
3) story telling

I've already mentioned the power of a killer playlist, so now you can remember the M in the seven-step process of E.M.P.A.T.H.Y. as Making decisions...can you also remember the E without looking?

Side note: I'm also a fan of action words – that is, words that end in -*ing*. Think is not the same as *thinking* and do is not the same as *doing*. See how often you can put action words into your thoughts, which helps bring them to life.

As in every chapter, let's dive into some knowledge that would be helpful. It's not necessarily that you don't already know what I'm sharing with you as much as, are you actively using/doing it? When it comes to making decisions, it's helpful to first evaluate the thought that preceded it. One of the best ways to do this is to ask questions like, "What was I thinking?" or "How did I come to that conclusion?" Are you ready?

Question: Do you know your body type? And I don't mean fat or skinny. There are basically three body types, just like there are types of hair and eye color, ranges of big boned and petite, and even whether you're musical or not. I so wish I had musical talent, but I'm not willing to "work" for it because I prefer to expand on what comes "naturally" to me. The same goes for body types. It's best to embrace what you've got and work with it! Like the gal with naturally curly hair who wishes it was straight, and the gal with straight hair who thinks it's boring. Why waste time wishing for what you don't have, or not appreciating what you do have - that others wish for – and instead, expand on your signature greatness?

This knowledge is helpful in making decisions about your plan of action because sometimes, we strive to be like someone from a different morph. Knowing your morph type allows you to stop going after what's not in your wheelhouse and focus more on making the best of what you've got. And girl, you've got a lot. Morph types are similar to the hair analogy in the fact that the one we have is often not the one we wish we did. And the one we have, is the one others wish they had - follow me?

The three body types I'm referring to are "morphs." And here they are in a nutshell...

1. Endomorph (the slow burner) - this body type has always struggled with keeping the weight off but is generally happier and healthier than the other morphs.

2. Ectomorph (the fast burner) - this is the body type that burns calories fast and has trouble keeping weight on. However, they are generally high-strung and very hard on themselves.

3. Mesomorph (the steady burner) - this is the body that, if they stay active, can maintain a healthy weight. But as soon as the activity wanes, the weight comes on – especially in the belly.

As you can see, each has their pros and cons, and it's possible that due to excessive dieting of some form during your pubescent years – or even after – you may have experienced all the morphs. However, you *intuitively* know which one you are - the one you relate to the most today.

With this knowledge, you can have more empathy for what you bring to the table in this life and how to make the best of it. Decide which one's best suit you now, take notes, and become more loving and kinder to the body you're in.

If you're the slow burner, endomorph, a good plan would include movement you love and awareness of when you choose food to help you forget your troubles. Embrace all the love and laughter that comes more easily to you in life. Get out of the house as much as possible.

If you're the fast burner, ectomorph, a good plan would include watching your refined sugar and caffeine intake. Just because you can, doesn't mean it's good for you. And appreciate that fat is not your problem. Find ways to live, love, and laugh more.

If you're the steady burner, mesomorph, a good plan would be to stay active! You're blessed with coordination and a body that loves to move – so give it what it wants and you'll both be happy. Find a good recreational league and start playing again.

This awareness allows you to hone in on what comes easily for you and to stop expecting different results from a body that's not designed for that journey.

At this point, you have a decision to make. Embrace your morph type* and celebrate all the good it also brings or continue to wish you were another. Either choice brings consequences for better or worse, because even inaction is a choice with consequences.

Next up is what to do about your environment. It's so easy to assume that "if only you hadn't..." things would be different. Hello! Are you still going all external on me? We're getting R.E.A.L. here and making a plan for lasting change. Unless you're going to just walk away from your family, spouse, job, or move, it's time to make a R.E.A.L. plan. I speak from experience when I say, "You can't run away from your troubles." So, here we go again with embracing what you love and adapting what's not so great into something possible that supports your health and happiness.

Do you think everyone who walks out on family, their career, marriage, relationships, or gets out of town is happy and healthy? Maybe? Does this sound like something you're *really* energized about? If yes, then make a plan and act on it! Stop blaming others for the reason why you are unhappy, overweight, and on meds. Just remember, who you are, and your happiness is an inside job that never finishes. It's always evolving, ideally onward and upward.

Here's your next assignment/opportunity: Write down the top three things you'd like to change about your life, the steps necessary, *and* the outcome you anticipate. Then look at how much of this you are passionately energized about and could make happen easily with just a bit of effort, because your passion and desire are so strong. Allow pleasure to motivate you.

Now, if you can't find anything you're so passionate about that you'd be willing to exert that much energy into making it manifest, then let's get back to baby steps. Pick one and just take the first step. See how successful and easy it was. Then continue to do *that* until it's part of who you are – how you think, feel, and act. Now you're on the path to a R.E.A.L. life. Celebrate what's working and accept what's not as just a bump in the road. If it's more of a pothole than bump, maybe it needs some attention and TLC. Only you know that answer.

Back in the day, when I was big into goals and affirmations, I decided I wanted a helicopter. I did this exact assignment. I sat down and made the list of why I wanted it and the steps necessary. Well, it didn't take long for me to see how way off I was in this decision. Once I got real energized about it, I realized it was not for me. The cost, storage, licensing, fuel, and insurance alone took away the glamor. Since then, I've just rented one – pilot and all of course – to get where I wanted to go. And guess what... that's only been twice in thirty years. The romance we choose to live in our heads about what we deserve can be very disheartening when compared to the action steps necessary that bring it from romance to real. That's why it's important to understand the difference between real and realistic desires. It's not that the helicopter was unrealistic, it was just not what I *really* wanted after it was out of my head and made real. Let me know if you need more clarity on this very important concept. It's the first step in the success of my coaching practice.

What's your first step? How are you making your life real instead of romantic? Romance is great, if it's based in reality. Just because I call Dwayne Johnson my boyfriend, put his name as my boyfriend in caller ID, and have an autographed picture of him on my mantle, it still doesn't make it real, just a romantic notion. Those are not actions that build a relationship. They only support the fantasy. Get real with actions that support your desires and make them happen for you – because you deserve it.

What are you going to do if you love where you live, but the winters are brutal and you always gain weight, get depressed, and wish you were somewhere else… until spring comes and you fall in love all over again? I can't answer that for you, but you can and will, if you really want to get happy and healthy and are no longer blaming your external situations.

What are you going to do if you hate your soul-sucking job? Do you quit, stay eighteen more years for retirement, find a way to remember that you're only there eight-ish hours a day and it does not define you? Or, do you want to follow your dream and become self-employed? Are you ready to give up vacation pay, insurance benefits, a reliable income, and getting out of the house every day? Maybe, maybe not. So, make that list and get real with yourself.

This assignment makes real what you want. And, when you get what you want, you become happier and healthier every day, more and more.

Bonus: When you're faced with a big decision,
"Take it to the board."

I use a guided meditation, where you close your eyes, take those bigger slower breaths, in and out, while putting your thoughts in the back seat for a minute or two, remembering to relax your shoulders down and away from your ears while expanding your belly and rib cage with each breath. Allow your exhalation to be twice as long as your inhalation. Then, imagine a boardroom table with you at the head, and your heart and gut on either side. Place no judgement on how this looks in your imagination. The visuals are just placeholders for the conversation.

Next, ask your question or state your dilemma to each of the three at the table. Listen without interrupting as each one gets its say – no matter how insane. After each of them have spoken, your brain/ego, heart/self-love, and gut/intuition, thank them for the wisdom they bring to the table. Then take all the time you need to slowly open your eyes and write down what you know now that was not clear before. Sometimes you will get conflicting messages, but the meditation is designed to help you get out of your own way and make a more informed decision. Very often your first step will be revealed. Try it...I believe you'll like it!

Let's review: The best way to start making R.E.A.L. good decisions is to stop blaming. Take control by writing out what you want, figure out why, and how to get it, and then get quiet while you relax into your body and listen to what it wants you to know. It loves you. Watch out for your ego telling you what you can't do and look instead toward the thoughts and actions of what's possible. Remember not to fantasize too much, yet still allow your hopes and desires to bubble up – they've been waiting.

The rules here are similar to that of the genie in the bottle...

1. No asking for more wishes. Work on three or less at a time.

2. You can't make someone fall in love with you, but you can fall back in love with yourself.

3. You can't bring someone back from the dead. Forget about the one that got away, or the mistake you think cost you your career. Live and learn now.

Making important decisions about how you know you can be living your life and how to make that possible is a daunting step. However, I believe you are still reading this book because you've had enough. You're fed up with life passing you by and too many other people - who aren't even happy or healthy - calling the shots for you.

This is a very good time to remember why you want and deserve this, as well as the fact it's a process, not a pill. Your positive decisions followed by supportive actions bring the results you have been longing for.

Ready to put the passion back into your life?

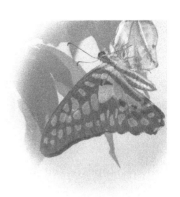

Chapter 6:

P – Prioritizing Your Passion!

Getting Clear on and in Touch with What Matters to You Most

What sparks passion and joy in your life? Do you even remember? If someone asked, what would you tell them? And would you be truthful?

Answer those questions from a place of unconditional love and benevolence to begin redesigning your life. Don't remember what unconditional love feels like? Well stop right now, close your eyes, and call out all the faces of people who have and will always love you – especially include the pets! Quit feeling sorry for yourself. Sorry people are not healthy people. If you are really going to try and tell me no one loves you, then I'll have to tell you to stop blocking the love. Yup, stop it! There's a hysterical YouTube video from the old TV show, Bob Newhart, called "Stop It". You have my permission to watch it *after* you finish this chapter – sure, I know you're going to it now, so just promise you'll come back with your highlighter in six minutes.

How about the million-dollar question: "Why are you here?" When you write the answer to this challenging question, I'll bet my honu* collection you don't write "to be fat, lazy and on meds." But the answer to that question often gets blocked by our ego, which can keep us from living our life on purpose with passion.

Now before I start sounding too metaphysical, I want to give you your next assignment (opportunity), which is not to be done until you finish the first round of this book so the answers will have more truth in them.

Spend as much time as you like writing down everything that "lights your fire." Your answers can be everything from "finding a penny heads-up on the ground" to "eating a meat lovers pizza with my son." The sky's the limit, no restrictions or judgement. Just fill page after page of people, places, things, events, and fantasies until you think you might be repeating yourself. You may even want to do this more than once during the week. It's good fun and starts to shift your mindset toward what's possible, because the list will mostly be things you've already enjoyed or are enjoying – which make them 100% possible! You are so unique and amazing, and this assignment will help remind you of that and more.

We all require different things to light our fire. My list, for example, would include giving a TED Talk and would never include fishing. Yet for many, giving a speech would make them terrified and fishing would be the best way to spend a nice day.

Here's what's happening. Due to high cortisol* your stress levels are directly related to your waistline. And since you *cannot physically* be stressed and in bliss at the same time, it's mandatory that you're going to start bringing back some of that blissful passion.

It makes sense that it's okay to be overweight and on meds because so many others are, and it's not your "fault," right? Wrong! It's like trying to turn right to get home because that's "safer" since you never have to cross traffic, even though your home is just three houses to the left and on the left side. So, guess what? If you took a left with more confidence, you'd be home sooner enjoying yourself.

Remember what I said earlier about why loved ones like you lumpy? Well, if you keep stressing each other out, you'll continue to be dangerously big around the midsection. We can thank Dr. Oz for bringing to our attention the dangers of visceral fat* aka: belly fat. If possible – and perhaps it's not – getting your loved ones to understand passion again will make your journey so enjoyable. What types of things are you passionate about together? Teamwork makes the dream work.

Next, let's get real about your relationship with time. The construct of time is literally just a figment of our imagination. Have you ever been waiting for a bus, for example, versus on the computer looking for flights to Hawaii? How do the same twenty minutes of time compare? Do they feel the same? After all, twenty minutes is the same no matter what, right? Of course not! When you have a better idea of how much power you actually have over your time – specifically your "free time" - you'll be able to have time for the things you love on that list that rock your world and bring passion back into your thoughts and actions.

At a glance, here is what a solo person's week can look like:

- Sleep
- Work
- Chores/Tasks
- Getting ready/Hygiene
- Commuting
- Cooking/Eating/Meal Prep

Now, write your own. Do your best to not pick out the *one* thing that's not right in the way your schedule looks. Just get the overall big picture and then adapt it for you. For example, if you work the night shift, have kids, don't have kids, work on the weekends, have two jobs or whatever, you'll need to adapt the schedule. Keep in mind that everyone has the same twenty-four hours in a day, but how they enjoy them is so very optional. You have choices, so choose to make changes, or figure out how to shift time in your favor.

Now you can see how even if you don't feel you can leave your well-paid, soul-sucking job, you can still have time for a passionate life when you remove the "mindless" activities like all non-work-related screen time. And trust me, passion burns calories like wildfire!

Screen time is the silent killer of your health, body, relationships, and brain functions. But you already know this. It's all about remembering you have the power, you make the decisions, so choose from a better mindset. In order to think better, you've got to first turn off the screens because *no*, you can't multitask. But you can do several things badly at once.

Remember the gal who quit her job to become a yoga instructor and nature guide? That could be you, in your own very special and one-of-a-kind awesome way.

Bring It!

Are you ready to say, "Bring It!"? I hope so because now it's time to identify your demons. I never said it was all going to be easy. If it were easy, no one would be overweight and on meds, right? Okay, are you for *real* ready? If yes, say "Bring It!" out loud like it's going to win you a million bucks! Because it's sure going to make you feel like it.

Here we go... take out that list of things that lights you up like a full moon on a clear night, and then (cue scary music), set a timer for ninety seconds and make a list of all the reasons why you can't really have all *that* any more. These are your demons and it's time to slay them.

Now, pick three of the easy ones you believe don't really have much power over you any more or not so much. Then make a plan to annihilate them – show them who's boss.

Here's an example: I love playing softball (passion) but I'm too fat and lazy to be any good anymore (demon). (Action) I'm going to join a recreational slow pitch co-ed softball team ASAP! This one alone will also slay the demon of not getting out of the house outside of work, making new friends, and the E word.

Another: I love playing chess (passion) but my brain has gone to mush, and no one likes a nerd (demons). (Action) I'm going to find or start a chess club! This kills two demons with one action because you came to slay!!! Not sure if you have the online group site called "Meetup"? It's an easy place to get started on so many activities. Or, start your own.

And one more, because we can work on three at a time, remember?

I love traveling (passion) but I can't afford it (demon). (Action) I'm making a jar to put money in every time I don't spend it on fast food or chain coffee. And while I'm saving, I'm going to look at all the affordable and interesting things to do in my own town. This is also a multi-slayer because it covers addressing your "bad" food habits, saving money, getting out of the house, *and* the E word. Once that jar gets full, put it in the savings. Find some pics to put up of where you'll be going.

This is how you prioritize your passion, stop wallowing in self-deprecation and get happy and healthy again. There's a lot of words in that last sentence that are worth looking up.

Side note: If you're still wondering what all this has to do with weight loss, well, let me tell you again. If you were drawn to this book because of the allure of not having to diet and exercise to get what you desire, then you surely knew that something was going to have to be different, and that you'd need to make some changes to get back your happy and healthy life. Right? Wonder no more. The answer is, you will be giving up all the old stories and misinformation that's been allowing you to stay stuck in an unhealthy state of mind and body.

I'd like to paraphrase a story here about how elephants are trained for captivity. Supposedly, when elephants are babies, they are tied to a heavy stake in the ground with a thick strong rope. While they are little, the stake and rope are too much for them to escape from. So over time they believe "escape" is not possible. By the time they are fully grown they could easily pull themselves free from the stake and rope, *however,* they don't believe it's possible.

I don't know why people would train fleas, but I heard the same story about that as well except it was the lid on a jar. Kind of reminds me of what we call today "the glass ceiling."

I'd like you to take a moment right now to reflect on where you may have been an elephant or a flea, trained into believing you can't ever be healthy and happy again. Journal it. Get it out of your head so you can look at it on paper and see *how limiting* it has been. Then claim your power to break free!

This is exactly how and why you have been drained of your passion and purpose in life. Who really cares if you take care of your body/temple? You should! When you have passion it's easier to wake up happy, because you have things to truly look forward to and get going on. The best way to find passion and put it into action is to actively seek it out, give it a big ol' hug, and make it your new best friend.

Bonus: Here's another, very easy Guided Meditation to help you connect with your purpose:

"What's my message for today?"

Begin with closing your eyes and relaxing your jaw and shoulders while you breathe those big, deep, long, and slow meaningful breaths that help your chatty brain to relax and join you on this journey into your imagination. Take as long as you like.

First, bring out the image that, just for today and this process, represents your higher power, your True Source, beyond your physical self (remember, no judgement on any of the images you see), then just relax and allow the unconditional love to flow to you and through you.

Next, see yourself looking at your higher power and ask the question, "What's my message for today?" After you get your message – and it could just be a feeling – take all your images back inside and slowly open your eyes. If you like the message, write it down. However, if it was mean, scornful, judgmental or angry, then don't. Your True Source will always be loving and kind in its communication with you. If it scolds or reprimands you, it will be very loving, not intimidating. Sometimes you may not get a message and that's okay, just enjoy the "reset" you got while relaxing through the process. And if your ego got in the way and pretended to be your higher power, with a chastising message, just tell it thanks for sharing but that's not the truth and you know it! Over time it gets easier to hear your True Source/Voice.

Let's review: Finding your passion is a lot like salsa dancing – one step forward, one back, cha cha up, cha cha back. Going back is not always a bad thing. Sometimes it gives you momentum (like a slingshot), which allows you to change direction, or just let life be what it is – yours. So, get real about how much time you're actually wasting every day, make your lists, pick the three you're confident you can master by slaying the demon and start living again, on your own terms, in line with where you are capable of being in your life right now. Because you are so capable and no longer a coward. You have lived in the shadows long enough. The time is now to allow yourself to live in the light because you are radiant, and your gifts and talents must shine.

And you now have time on your side. If you feel there are too many to slay at once, that's okay because you understand time is on your side. Just do what feels possible from a place of passion and be tenacious – hang in there through the hiccups. If it was always smooth sailing it would be so boring – you know that.

Now, let's go from sloth to superstar!

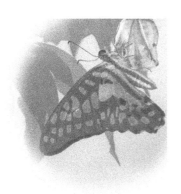

Chapter 7:

A – ACTUALLY DOING IT!

Why Most People Are All Talk and No Action

Are you ready to go from sloth to superstar? Really? You know that means making changes and going from wishing to willing – so, are you really, ready? I believe you are, simply because you're still here.

This is the chapter where you understand why motivation is like caffeine, as well as how to stay self-reliant through the lows, and on-course during the distractions of the highs.

Are you getting used to using and thinking in "-ing" words yet? We learned that in chapter five on making decisions. This one simple step will be a cornerstone for success in the long run. You will continue to think and do things that are supporting your *true* self by acting in a way that you know is for your greater good. Sound good? Alrighty then, let's just do it!

Think like Tigger, even if you're feeling more like Eeyore or Rabbit, and watch the transformation unfold right before your eyes. Try this...

Which of the following statements "feels" better when you say them out loud or in your head?

I have to drive the kids to school early tomorrow.
I'm driving the kids to school early tomorrow.

The first one is more of a mandated chore, where the second is a choice. If you honestly don't feel a difference, that's okay. You're just new to this action feeling thing. Once you get the hang of it, it will become second nature and you'll begin to notice what a bummer those "bossy" statements sound like. Here's another example:

I turn fifty this year.
This year, I'm turning fifty.

Again, the first one is a mandate that gives no feeling of control, where the second, feels a little exciting. Third one's a charm...

I have to go to Zumba tonight.

Or, I can't miss my Zumba class tonight.

I'm looking forward to going to Zumba tonight.

The last statement not only has a positive feeling embedded in it, but two action words, making it very powerful. This is one of many techniques used in Neuro Linguistic Programming (NLP)*

I know I said earlier I'm not a fan of affirmations and here's why: they generally don't baby-step, so your mind laughs the affirmation off as a joke rather than a statement of fact.

When you make the affirmation, "I no longer eat fast food," your brain/ego laughs, and says, "Who are you talking about?" A baby step would be, "Now I'm only eating the kids meals at fast food joints." See how that can be something possible, a good place to start – a baby step. Over time you can move up to, "The only fast food I eat any more is (fill in the blank)," which then becomes, "I don't enjoy eating fast food," to which your brain will then say, "I know, right."

I've always been fascinated by words and as a kid was known as a "bookworm." So, when I was exposed to NLP, I dove right in and became a certified practitioner. It's still my number one favorite keynote presentation.

I'm going to give you just a few pieces of the tip of the NLP iceberg so you can have lasting success in your weight management and overall wellness.

The first one is the power of the action, "-ing" verb words; the second is the embedded command or presumption. This is not to be confused with an assumption – let me explain...

Presumption: an idea that is taken to be true, and often used as the basis for other ideas, although it is not known for certain.

Assumption: a thing that is accepted as true or as certain to happen, without proof.

Although they may sound similar, the power is in presumption because it is malleable. It can evolve and take on other shapes and forms, which makes it easier for your mind to accept. Whereas assumption is perceived as more of a fact, where the mind can argue rather than adapt. If you still don't see a difference, it's because I'm a word nerd and you don't have to highlight this section. No worries, because there's plenty of good stuff to be putting into action already.

Here are a few embedded commands with presumption.

- I'm signing up at the yoga studio after work today – Yay me! Anyone joining me?
- I'm having a fancy salad for dinner to mix things up. I'm actually looking forward to it.
- I'm taking the TV out of my bedroom tonight because I'm tired of being tired and wasting time in bed – Yay me again. (Now I'm thinking of all the other things I can be doing in bed instead!)

You get the idea. When you're writing three of your own to be working on from your passion list, remember to pick the ones you believe you'll have the most success with. Or, jump in the deep end and pick one that you currently have the most desire for. You can also pick just one and write three supporting actions for it.

Ready for another piece of eye-opening NLP advice? When talking to yourself, do your best to avoid negative words like "can't," "won't," "don't," and Universal Qualifiers (UQ's) like "always" and "never." Why? Great question. Because believe it or not, your brain is positively positive. That means creation comes easily where destruction is harder. If I say, "Close your eyes and don't picture a pepperoni pizza." Bam! There it is, manifested instantly in your imagination because your mind is meant for creation. Then, you can take the image away, but it takes more effort and can only be done after the fact. I beg you to please highlight this section! Say what you want, not what you don't. Think about what happens when you tell your kids, or yourself, that they can't have or do something.

It's challenging in the beginning and it's crucial that you support your awareness in this area of your thoughts. If you find your thoughts to be non-stop negative, applaud your *awareness* because now you can make changes. You must first be aware there is a "problem" before you can take action to correct it.

Okay, so what's up with the UQ's? Going forward, every time you hear yourself say "never," "always," "everyone," "no one," and "every time," follow that up with the single UQ question.

Examples:

- I'm always going to be fat. Always?
- I'm never going to get in shape. Never?
- Everyone talks about me behind my back. Everyone?

How is this helpful? The idea here is to stop making assumptions and pull yourself out of the pity party. It's pretty easy once you become aware. And I'll bet you'll even enjoy this process. I often laugh when I correct myself.

Here's an example that happens to be a true story: My adult daughters laugh about it now and have shared appreciation for what they know today. But when they were younger, they got so frustrated (and frustrated is a kind word here) when I would challenge their UQ language. And boy, do teenagers use a ton of UQ's.

It's a great conversation starter! Here is an example: Teen says, "Everyone thinks I'm ugly!" Mom says, "Now honey, you always know I think you're beautiful. I'll bet they're just jealous." Teen slams the door to their room, "Mom you don't know anything!"

Here is how it can go: Teen says, "Everyone thinks I'm ugly!" Mom says, "Everyone?" Teen says, "Well not *everyone,*" and rolls her eyes, "just the popular guys."

Now you have just earned yourself an open-door conversation. When you have better thoughts and communication with yourself and others, you begin to reduce stress. When you reduce stress, you don't seek comfort food, TV, and alcohol as a way to "handle it." Less stress means more oxygen to your brain which leads to better decision making.

The ability to make better decisions, rather than self-medicating into avoidance is the best way to eliminate stress in the first place – before it settles in and becomes dis-ease. It takes some practice, but not as much as you think, once you remind the ego that you're making the decisions. Happy and healthy are just one good thought after another away - for starters.

Recently, one of my clients wanted to know how "negative" her website was, so we went through it, page by page, and found over one-hundred instances where she misdirected, confused, or negated the sales and information. I'll just give you one – "Don't miss out on the monthly newsletter." What you want to say is... "Ready for all the tips and hacks only the insiders know?" Create urgency! Begin with the voices in your head, so you can start being more effective and positive in your actions.

Bonus: I know that may be a lot to digest so let me give you a few more Webster definitions to help you move along more quickly in understanding why goals and affirmations have failed you.

Affirmation: "Emotional support or encouragement." This is the second definition in the dictionary because the first on uses the word in the definition – ugh, that's not helpful.

Affirmations fail you because until they "feel" true, nothing will come of it or at least stick around long-term once those old thoughts worm their way back again. If you have the power to put passion and a great visualization with them, you've got a fighting chance they'll come true. Most folks just want to believe if you say it enough, you'll begin to believe it. Again, saying is not as powerful as doing. Words are not enough and that's why you failed.

Goal: "The object of a person's ambition or effort; an aim or desired result." Since we're not talking sports (which was the first definition) this second definition is also more applicable and there is that word desire again.

The reason goals have failed you is most likely because they were just words, or something that would be "nice" to accomplish. But, when it came time to put the pedal to the metal, the fun went out of it and so did your passion. I am a fan of goals when they are followed up with the right action and have flexibility. Goals work so much better with an accountability partner or coach. But you guessed it, not many take that crucial step.

Motivation: "The general desire or willingness of someone to do something." Again, I chose the second definition because of the words desire and willingness.

This is why I compare motivation to caffeine. It's all exciting, until it's not. Desire and willingness are adventurous traits that they don't teach us in school. Staying the course through thick and thin means digging deep and unearthing your champion. And who really likes to get dirty? Motivation is a tool best used for special circumstances – otherwise, your greatest tool is…

Action: "The fact or process of doing something, typically to achieve an aim." First choice definition because it totally defines this chapter – Doing!

I'm not going to pick on this one. Action is something we have the power to do. It goes wrong when we choose inaction, usually due to fear. Inaction is also an action in disguise.

Self: "A person's particular nature or personality; the qualities that make a person individual or unique. One's own power and resources."

I *love* this! Back to the question, "Who are you?"

Reliance: "Trust in someone or something."

Combine this with Self and now you've got a fighting chance. That's why prayer and meditation are so powerful, and why you've had such a tough time sticking to something in the past. You forget you're connected to a greater power, your True Source that's got your back if you would only trust. Self-reliance is a back-pocket superpower that we all possess.

Discipline: "The practice of training people to obey rules or a code of behavior, using punishment to correct disobedience."

Well now, can you see why your self-discipline wanes? What a horrible way to live. To all you disciplinarians out there, and "Please don't shoot!" I'm only asking that you compare the long-term success rate of self-discipline to self-reliance. Meditate on it.

Let's review: This, my friends, is how you go from sloth to super-star! Start with bringing action into your thoughts, followed by saying what you want versus what you don't, and supported by taking the power out of UQ's.

Things become possible when they become more fluid than fact. Your words come from your thoughts. Start thinking the way healthy people do and watch what comes out of (and goes into) your mouth. Take a fun journey into this by watching Simon Pegg's wild adventures in the movie *Hector and the Pursuit of Happiness.*

Bonus: In the Thank You section of this book, I'm providing a link to the article on "Why Motivation is like caffeine – and what you can do about it."

I think you're ready for the secret ingredient!

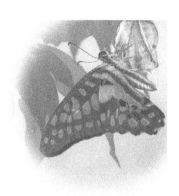

Chapter 8:

T – Thinking Your Way Back to a Body You Love

Why It's Never Been about Diet and Exercise (Or Pills)

This chapter is all about how to take back control and stand confidently in your decisions for better health, all while moving forward, and only backward when you feel off track. When you get good thoughts in place, everything else just falls in order or away. Things you enjoy show up more in your life and things that irritate or keep you down seem to miraculously fall away. Don't believe me? That's because you have not been aware of how the process of *Thoughts, Emotions, and Actions* impact your reality.

How is this possible? It's because now, you understand how to create the life/body you desire and are also willing to take the baby steps (or leaps) necessary. Before, you were so tethered to your past (much like the elephant in chapter six), how people treated you, and your circumstances, that you did not see *how* they were stepping-stones to your lack of success.

I'm so excited I'm ready to burst! Let's get started on this information (and get that highlighter!)

You may have said, "I don't know what I was thinking?" while in reality, every action is the *final* step in making your choices. First there is always a thought. Sometimes it's a voice or faint whisper in your head, like, "I'll show them who's in charge of my eating!" Then that thought creates an emotion, like anger, resentment, or frustration. Then, that emotion leads you to take action. But remember, inaction is also a choice. Like when you make bad food choices instead of what you intended - or claimed you intended - to eat.

Please highlight! Your actions are fueled by your emotions, so it makes sense that negative emotions lead to poor choices for action. For example, if you're feeling resentful, it's much less likely you'll do something nice for someone or yourself. I've never said, "Man, it was a tough day. I can't wait to get home and have a big salad." You get the idea. It's pretty basic, yet most folks don't want to believe that most everything is in their control, or even worse, the thought that anything "bad" in their lives was brought on by themselves. Blame is so much easier, and even sometimes fun, compared to taking responsibility and checking your thoughts around the origin of what went down after the fact.

It's worth restating; actions are always preceded by your thoughts - no exceptions. The sooner you develop the skill of getting back to the root of your actions by asking yourself, "What was I feeling before I did/didn't do that?" Followed by, "And what was I thinking that triggered that emotion?" You'll soon be able to take control and change those thoughts into healthier, more loving, kind, and supportive ones. That means you being happier, fitter, and off the meds easier!

Another highlightable moment; happy thoughts keep you healthier in your emotions and actions. Happy people are rarely sick because dis-ease can't settle in and make a home. This is *exactly* why I've been shouting from the rooftops for all who are ready to embrace this concept: you can be overweight and off the meds. Not extremely obese, but much heavier than that *magic number*. Only you can create your magic, and it is different for everyone.

A six-foot athlete can weigh so much more than a six-foot deconditioned person, without the side effects of snoring, sleeplessness, loss of libido and such. That makes sense, right? Take some time and think about what your personal magic number could be. It can and will change with the ebb and flow of life. But for now, pick your first-round number. Make sure it's doable and motivational enough to get there with baby steps (or leaps of faith) you are so ready and willing to make.

True story: I'm a second-hand survivor of domestic violence. When I was fourteen, I was invited to sit in with my mom at one of her counseling sessions. I was off the charts proud of my mom for reaching out for professional help and was bouncing in my chair in the waiting room. Well, in a nutshell, the counselor began to explain to us that the first step in making change for our situation was for my mom to see how she was fueling the violence. *What*? My mom was the victim, not the perpetrator! I was so furious I wanted to strangle that man right where he sat, so calm and smug-like. Um, perpetuating violence? But of course, I just stuffed my emotions with a smile and nod, pretending nothing was crazy wrong - like I'd been doing for the last decade. I told my mom the guy was an idiot who obviously had never been traumatized and that she should never go back.

Fast-forward ten years, and I discover the knowledge that we are here to grow and play a big role in that learning. In hindsight, I would never in a million years say my mother deserved to be beaten. What I'm hoping you will understand, like we both did, was there were things that could have been different. Awareness of your thoughts leads to the ability to affect change. While you are the "victim" you cannot see how to "escape" and get to freedom. Outsmart the oppression by remembering that you have a purpose, and it's not to be suppressed by a bully.

All righty then, enough talk and theory. Let's review your *Thoughts, Emotions*, and *Actions,* so you can practice *how* to become brave and take the actions necessary for your overall health and happiness. Remember, just like doctors and attorneys *practice* their craft, so will you cultivate the ideal thoughts for you at this moment in time. As you grow, you may adapt this as you experience other situations which help you also cultivate this craft. Kind of like how some people start drinking coffee with tons of cream and sugar, then adapt to just black – or not.

Step one is to become aware of your thoughts about what's happening. Then decide what you want/deserve and make a plan. Basically, awareness of your thoughts pulls them into the light for you to decide which ones are worthy of the life you are here to live.

All of that begins to explain your next step of emotions. Allow your emotions to be sign-posts. They are not the end-all, simply a bonus for your awareness. If you missed the thought, your emotions are your next fail-safe to get your course corrected. I'd put my Domo collection up on eBay if you told me you prefer to be angry, frustrated, or sad. That's how positive I am that you really prefer to be happy. That's not to say that every day will be a perfect day full of sunshine and rainbows. Of course, you know that.

Your emotions can be so powerful that they magnify your thoughts and the next thing you know it's, "What was I thinking?" Saying sorry sucks and losing weight is a physical expression of apologizing to your body. Emotional eating is where this all hangs in the balance.

The last step is action, and that can only happen when you choose *awareness*. Things can't change if you choose not to look at them for what they really are...Thoughts, Emotions, and Actions. You may not feel like you have control over your thoughts at first because you have not attempted to be the leader in a very long time. Have you ever told a four-year-old to do something and they just flat out told you, "No"? Ah, the good old days when we were large and in charge. Let's get back to the power of a toddler and remember, we can say "no", especially when it supports our greater good and overall happiness.

Ever get cut off in traffic and are forced to slam on your brakes to make room for the idiot? Well, I'd imagine - from experience - you think you felt angry. However, you actually *first* had a thought. And that thought led to how you then reacted (Emotion + Action). So, what if you rolled up next to the idiot to give them a piece of your mind and they apologized, saying their wife just left work in labor after her water broke. Would your Thoughts, Emotions, and Actions change? If your answer is "no," we need to chat ASAP.

I really despise the term "comfort food." It implies something warm and fuzzy. Binge eating comfort foods is your way of saying, "I didn't like my thoughts, which made me feel (fill in the blank), so I'll just avoid the whole problem by stuffing my face until I fall asleep. Then if my thoughts wake me, I'll just eat some more until I feel better." Well, that's an ugly scenario! And you know it but are choosing to do nothing about it. Need I remind you? Inaction is also an action.

"Wait!" I can hear some of you saying. "I like comfort food and I'm not going to give it up!"

Who said you had to give it up? Why are you trying to fail the process? All you need to do, toddler style, is to remember that you know what makes you happy. And then, adult style, moderate what is not good for you just because you "feel like it". Emotions/feelings are the second step, so if you're feeling something, it's your responsibility to pause and go back a step to the first step, thought. Analyze that thought and the message it brings so you can feel better about it and take a more supportive action.

Understanding and implementing these processes in the order defined, I believe, is the most powerful information you never been allowed to know.

Can we get nerdy for a moment? The Habenula*

There are journals full of research and documentation on the little, teeny, teensy, weensy piece of your brain known as the habenula. Here it is in a nutshell, so you can understand how you've gotten in the situation you're in and that you also have the power to make change.

Thriving in a world with hidden rewards and dangers requires choosing the appropriate behaviors or you'll just be surviving. Recent discoveries indicate that the habenula plays a prominent role in these choices through the reward motivated behavior (dopamine) and happy behavior (serotonin) systems. Moreover, the habenula is involved in behavioral responses to pain, stress, anxiety, sleep and reward, and its dysfunction is associated with depression, schizophrenia, and drug-induced psychosis. Yikes! As a highly conserved structure in the brain, the habenula provides a fundamental mechanism for both survival and decision-making.

Are you still awake? I said it was nerdy. I just wanted to give you the science behind the actual mental, emotional, and physical basis you have as a human for your future success.

The good news is, the habenula is adaptable - what was, is not what *has to be* forever. Reward-based decision-making can affect positive thoughts. Now the catch here is if you reward your "bad" behavior, you'll continue to make bad decisions. However, you can choose to reward your "good" behaviors and release the dopamine that supports your happiness.

Here's an example: When you choose fast food over and over even though you know it's not healthy, then allow yourself to feel good or even okay about it, you train your habenula to allow you to feel *good* about a *bad* action. However, going forward, every time you choose fast food, don't beat yourself up, but do have a lot of internal discussion about why you chose fast food, what other options you really had, and how you can make a better choice next time. Then, really be mindful about how you feel physically after a non-nutritious meal. Basically, you're putting that action on notice as not so *good* anymore.

Avoidance of punishment is another area that needs to be addressed when it comes to the habenula. Not addressing something until the stress of it causes so much pain that you may act drastically is something to be hyper-aware of. Stress tells the habenula to shut down action and resort to the "deer in the headlights" of non-action, not wanting to move or make good choices. This also takes the form of procrastination.

Understanding the reward/punishment process of the habenula is another crucial step in your journey to a life that is happier, fitter, and off the meds. This time I'll wager my Korbel winery club membership that you were never enlightened about this process. Why? Because this knowledge gives you back your power and the ability to change your circumstances on a dime. Some habits may take a bit longer to improve, but not as long as they took to develop, once you become aware.

It's interesting how homeostasis will allow us to keep doing something we know is "bad" for us while keeping us from shifting to thoughts and actions we are confident can and will improve our quality of life. Hmm…time to get serious about that habenula!

Overview: Like I said before, do you want to be motivated by pleasure or pain? The choice is yours. They both lead to results. You have the power to reward yourself with happiness.

Begin by being aware of the voices in your head and hearing their language. Who is your highest power: your ego, or your subconscious? Once you have your thoughts on your radar for awareness, then you have more control over your emotions and actions. Especially going forward in life.

Once you have your thoughts on your radar/awareness, then you have more control over your emotions and actions. To delve deeper into that subject, go to www.truespeak.us and receive a free e-book entitled *The Positive Purpose of Negative Emotions* which guides you through the process of transforming your negative thoughts and emotions.

This is the secret ingredient, my friends, to achieving all you desire. Not a piece of cake, but more the recipe to create the results you deserve. Start at the root. Treat the cause not the symptom. Become mindful of *not* what goes in your mouth, but in your mind.

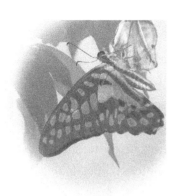

Chapter 9:

H – HAPPINESS: THE BEST DIET EVER!

It's off the Charts Good for You and Calorie Free

This chapter as all about learning what happiness looks, sounds, and feels like.

When you discover your path to daily happiness and learn to love the body you're in, it's a simple glide into a body that loves you back. Forget about weight loss and focus on putting your energy (aka: calories) into making your happiness first for the greater good!

Earlier we talked about the chaos theory and how to embrace the roller coaster ride that is life. No one makes it through without heartache, loss, disappointment, or rejection in some shape or form. Remembering this will be another cornerstone in the long-term success of your happiness. Because Happy = Healthy, you must understand why happiness is much more important to your overall wellness than anything else you spend your energy on.

Happiness, just like grumpiness, creates a butterfly effect that goes beyond that first action. First, let's talk about happiness. A while back, I was buying cosmetics and the lovely gal behind the counter asked for some wellness advice - she was overweight. I shared with her the most simple and successful tip I know: "Put on the shoes!" What that means is, when you put on the shoes that are specific to fitness (walking/running/workout), it tells your brain and body, "I'm getting ready to get moving!" Even if you manage to get on the shoes and sit back down to do something so very unsupportive to your wellness, your brain will keep on reminding you, "You put the shoes on!" It reminds of what happens when you pick up the leash for a walk but then sit back down in front of the T.V. There's no way, once you've chosen that one action of picking up the leash that the dog will let you forget it! Finally, you'll either choose to lose and never get moving. Or, you'll choose to live and get going.

Eight months later I saw the same gal again and she remembered me. She was so excited to tell me that she had lost twelve pounds just from that one simple act. She was so grateful to see me again to share her success. And she said she got other family members and her roommate to do the same! Ripple, ripple, flutter, flutter.

This is a perfect example of how *thinking* about doing something leads to much greater happiness when you *choose* to act on it and make it happen. The physical act empowers you and is sure to put a smile on your face out of sheer pride for yourself. It tells your body in an energetic and fun way, "Si, se puede!" (Yes, we can!)

Sadly, grumpiness works the same way. I'm going to paraphrase a popular story about "kicking the dog." Basically, this guy gets yelled at by his boss (who was grumpy), and then he yells at his associate (which made her grumpy), and then they all took it out on two or three others throughout the day (spreading grumpiness). Then, when they all got home, they yelled at and kicked their dogs. Ripple, ripple, flutter, flutter, in a "bad" way. The story then goes on to say, wouldn't it have been better to just start the day off kicking the dog - save all the grumpiness? Of course not! The point is, when you feel something trying to make you grumpy, just imagine the ripple effect of all those poor dogs getting kicked and shift the ripple. Because you can! It just takes awareness of your thoughts, which led to the emotion (grumpy), that led to the action (taking it out on the defenseless dog who loves you so unconditionally).

So how does this apply to you? Happiness is there for you in abundance when you use your secret ingredient everywhere you go. Now, let's get into some habits that will support you on your quest for happiness. I have hundreds of them, so am just going to share a few to get you started. This way you can pick the one(s) you like and put them into action ASAP and toss the one(s) you don't aside if they don't call to you.

Here's some more good news, forget that rule of sticking with just three actions I told you to follow earlier. When it comes to happiness, you get to create as much as you like. Be aware that when you begin this "diet" of happy thoughts, feelings, and actions, not everyone is going to like it. That's just fine, keep thinking of all the adorable doggies out there you are saving.

First, create a "Happiness" notebook. Record as much as you can in there for ninety days. The sky's the limit - Yay! Do your best to carry it with you and write in it often and faithfully. At minimum, after work to help reset you for home, or at bed to help you get a better night's rest. However, as often as possible is the goal. If you don't have your notebook (which is only for the happiness stuff) with you at the moment, then just say it out loud.

I enjoy saying "thank you" when I get green lights. It may sound silly but it's really very fun and a mood changer. What do I say at red lights? Nothing, I just start singing louder or practicing my foreign language. After ninety days (and mark it on the calendar), you can keep it up if it feels right or you can just do it once or twice a day. You will soon notice how easy it is to shift your mood when your thoughts are happy focused. Happy people are healthy people because the low vibration of dis-ease has nothing to match with. Simply put, stay hi-vibe.

A Happiness notebook is different from a gratitude journal in that the Happiness journal is designed to help you train the habenula for rewards on good thoughts and behaviors. This is possible because emotion is the language of the habenula. The Happiness notebook is for actions that make you laugh and smile, support healthy thoughts and actions, and assist in creating awareness on rewarding those events every time they happen, over and over again until they are just how you roll. Whereas, a gratitude journal is more for keeping your vibration hi-vibe as you recall things big and small to be grateful for that are currently in your life or memories. Shoes always make both lists for me – yes always.

Want a challenging one? Start complimenting yourself every single time you see your reflection. If it's hard to say, "you are one sexy babe," then just start by saying, "I am so lovable." If it's your mirror, look yourself in the eyes and say it with true passion. If it's a reflection, like in a window, say "I love you." This can be in your head or out loud.

Now take this one step further and start complimenting others - especially loved ones because we often get complacent and think they "just know" how wonderful we think they are. Then, ripple, ripple, flutter, flutter, and compliment strangers. It can be as simple as, "your nails are beautiful," to "I love that hairstyle on you." I recently told a young lady how radiant her smile was, and she immediately covered her mouth and said, "thank you." So, I followed that with "keep letting it shine, the world needs more smiles."

Here's a fun opportunity. Close your eyes and get into that nice state where you take deep and meaningful breaths that allow your brain to relax and slow down. Especially relax your jaw, shoulders, and belly as you breathe and put your focus there. And when you're ready, think about a funny story. Something you experienced that was not so funny at the time, but when you shared the story, everyone was laughing (yes, even you). Allow the laughter to wash over you until you're laughing out loud. Relive as many as you like. This is a great state changer that can be accomplished most any place or time.

Remember when you made that passion list? Get it out and look for something you can do in an instant.

And one more, even though it can get you in trouble. Go online and search for jokes. Write the best ones down and share them with others. Be the person who instead of gossips at the water cooler, tells the jokes. Watch people begin to count on you for the simple one-liners and even seek you out if they missed your joke of the day. I include jokes in all my virtual coaching. How can this get you in trouble? Anytime you go online searching for something random, you "lose" time. We talked about this already. So, maybe set a timer for three minutes or less and be prepared to write them down. I shouldn't have to remind you - avoid the dirty and rude ones.

Since we're talking about being online, go ahead and search baby anything. (Anything? Okay, most anything. You got me there.) Baby sloths, penguins, pandas, kittens, puppies and the like. If that doesn't put some happiness on your face and in your heart, we need to chat pronto.

Now let's talk about how happiness sounds. Of course, music is the best place to start! Remember the assignment earlier - no negative or harsh language lyrics for ninety days. Immerse yourself in sounds and music that soothes your soul and create a sense of happiness. Everyone is different. I personally don't care much for classical music or violins but to others, it's so beautiful. I enjoy funky disco music, which makes some folks grumpy. Mix it up, have fun, and let the music move you. This will also "magically" burn calories with all that extra foot tapping, singing, smiling, and such. You get the idea. After ninety days, I believe you'll find you may still like your "harsh" songs, but your tolerance will be lower. You will find yourself not liking some of the songs and hopefully you'll choose to stop listening to them all together.

Your language is another way to hear how happiness sounds. Remember to be choosing action words and asking for (and expecting) what you desire instead of what you don't. "Remember your lunch" is way better than "don't forget your lunch," because of how the brain processes information.

How does happiness look? It, like all the other components we've discussed, looks different to everyone – yes, everyone (this UQ is accurate). Happiness can look like volunteering, playing games, camping, painting, karaoke, and so on. Again, refer to your passion list for ideas and then work on making them happen so you can share that passion with others. Some people like running and they want me to join in on their passion, so I politely decline and encourage them to go for it! Happiness is a side effect of healthy - or is healthy a side effect of happiness? Either way, you'll notice the happier you are, the healthier you are. Go ahead and chant it! Happy = Healthy

Just to state the obvious, happiness also looks like a smile! Jeez, do I have to tell you that? Are you smiling now? Train the muscles in your face to make a slight, coy smile like you're up to something or know a secret. It's the simple effort of pulling up the corners of your mouth just a bit. Try it now, it's easy to do but if you haven't been doing it for decades, you'll really feel the muscles working. A slight smile travels all the way up to your eyes, making them sparkle, then it travels into your brain because if you're smiling, you must be happy. If you're concerned smiling will wrinkle your eyes and bring about crow's feet, then don't do it. Keep on with what you're doing and watch the sagging jowls of unhappiness hang from your jaw and affect your mindset. Again, with the choices. And of course, if you really want a radiant day, smile *big* and often. Whew, that's a workout. I also like to get as much laughter into my day as possible. It's a great way to get a smile on your face and laughing is an awesome ab workout! Remember, a smile is universal. No matter what country you're in, a smile means "happy" (or you're up to something that makes you happy).

True story: My mom is - according to the charts - obese. Yet her bloodwork shows healthy numbers. She is seventy-seven and her doctor tells her every year that she is her only patient in that age range who is not on any meds for being "obese." How is this possible? She is happy. In her retirement, she and her hubby volunteer, are in a car club, travel, and get out. She also works part-time and spends hours in her garden and going out with friends. A while back she slipped in the shower. Except for some ugly bruises, the x-rays showed no damage and her doctor commented that the "cushion" on her hips helped. So, there you go. And there are thousands of people just like her.

How can you be happy when there is so much to worry about and stress over? Remind yourself, the choice is yours. It's a perception. One person's fear is another's fantasy – remember, mine's doing a TED Talk, but how does that make you *feel*? Don't get all grumpy on me here...I understand that it's challenging to be happy when the car breaks down, you have the flu, or the in-laws come to stay for a spell. I am *not* saying you're going to be happy every second of every day. What I am saying with passion is, that if you are overweight and unhealthy, you need more happiness in your life. Happiness is an amazing drug you create, control the dosage, and the side effects are nothing short of miraculous. Happy people are healthy people because they avoid dis-ease. They can go with the tide instead of fighting the current. How? By remembering that there is so very much to be happy about! That's exactly why you've created your Happiness journal and write in it often.

Try this - walk around the room right now and literally touch everything you are grateful for. Yes, everything. Think about why it matters and what would happen if it got taken away suddenly. Make two or three columns in your Happiness Notebook and take three minutes to brainstorm everything you have for which you are so grateful. Sometimes, just for fun and to change my state, I'll exclaim "YAY" and clap my hands when the lights turn on, the water runs hot, or my toaster oven works. Fact: Not all people have these wonderful things to be happy and grateful in their lives – millions actually.

Now say for example, you hate your lumpy old couch. Well then, it's not going on the list. However, instead of feeling all grumpy about it, go buy or get a new one. Can't afford it? Try Facebook Marketplace or the Salvation Army (they have amazing stuff for a great price). Still can't afford it? Then just be glad you have it or you'd have to sit on the floor. That's a reframe.

If you are unhappy about something, someone, or a situation, then own it and make a plan for change and if you honestly want to say you have no control, then just embrace it and say, "Well, it is what it is for now." It will pass, lessons will be learned, you will survive - you have already survived so much. Create thoughts that are grateful and watch abundance flow to you so you can stop chasing it. Stop being the victim and begin acting like the rock star that you are - let your radiant-self shine!

Ripple, ripple, flutter, flutter. One of the best ways to do this is to volunteer. Don't have time? Take a solid look at the things you are spending time on that do not support your healthy mindset and stop doing them!! Your time is yours to create. There is nothing you *have to* do. Every action or inaction you take is your choice.

You don't *have to* go to work - lots of people either don't or wish they had a job to go to.

You don't *have to* do the laundry - some folks pay to have theirs done and some just wear it stinky.

You don't *have to* go to the bank at lunch – many people wish they money in the bank. Or even a lunch break, which means a job.

When doing chores, get happy by putting on a killer playlist and remembering that you have chores because you have these wonderful things like a home, clothes, food, and bathroom - for starters. Reframe your thoughts and this time, build something wonderful to live in. Stop letting your "have to's" weigh you down like rocks in the backpack you're choosing to wear.

Let's review: Happiness is a 100% *inside job* that will go a long way in your overall good health and wellness. It may be a bit challenging at first, but soon you'll feel the benefits and understand how your past perceptions created dis-ease in your life. Get out and experience all the free things in your own backyard, neighborhood, city, and state. Get some fresh air into your body and sunshine in your bones. Make the notebook, say thanks, compliment, smile, speak in words that are loving and kind, play that awesome playlist, volunteer, and remind yourself that you are literally a walking, talking, breathing miracle. If you're still not sold on the happiness thing, I give you permission to read Dr Andrew Weil's book, *Spontaneous Happiness*. It's so very refreshing – even for grumpy people.

Amen, and so it is!

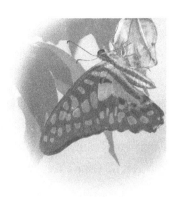

Chapter 10:

Y – YESTERDAY IS GONE FOREVER

Lessons Learned and Illusions Uncovered

As we evolve into the E.M.P.A.T.H.Y. Way, I hope you're getting the solid understanding of why I said earlier you could lose weight and get off the meds without diet and exercise. I never said anything close to you could stay on the couch, continue to eat junk, and never do anything physical. Happy = Healthy, plain and simple. There are tons of skinny people out there that are also unhealthy and on meds. It's worth repeating. I'm not a physician, nurse, or dietician, because this book is not about losing weight. It's about getting healthy; mentally and emotionally. I am a coach, mentor, and 30 plus year fitness professional. That's how I *know* this can work for you.

Yesterday is gone, and you'll see it when you *feel* it, *not* when you believe it are so closely related and yet a different part of your success.

The concept of letting go of yesterday is a biggie. For many, it's hard to truly grasp the idea that everything you have experienced in your past, for better or worse, is now just an illusion.

You have the power to keep the memories you enjoy and the ones that support your healthy mindset, and more importantly, let go of the ones that keep you tethered to dis-ease. Remember the elephant story? Here's how you do it. First, close your eyes and get into that nice state of deep and meaningful breaths, relaxing your jaw, shoulders, and belly. Then, call up a pleasant memory. While it's in your mind, allow yourself to connect with the good emotions which were part of that memory. As you recall it in the movie of your mind, enhance it. Make it more vivid in color, sound and depth. Feel yourself 3-D-like in the movie. Do this anytime you need a mental pick me up and reframe of your emotional state. Really *feel* how wonderful the experience was for you.

Now, do just the opposite with an old "bad" memory. Instead of connecting to the feelings (even though they may come up), do your best just to watch it and see your role in it as well as what it taught you. Then, play it again, but this time mess up the sound, the brightness, and fade yourself out of it. Hear the dialogue get garbled, watch it like the film is melting. If this is challenging, then make it funny. Put everyone in clown shoes and red noses, hear everyone with a helium voice and pitching back and forth like on a rocky boat at sea. This process allows you to "scratch" the memory so when it plays again, it won't have as much clarity or energy. Old school reference: like how if your record got warped or scratched – no matter how much you liked it – it never played the same again.

Another mandatory highlightable moment: Now that you understand the basics of NLP, this technique is easy to do and very effective. You'll know you've been successful when you can *remember* the memory, but no longer feel the negative emotion attached to it. How is this possible? Because you have learned the lesson. I can now talk about crazy stuff that happened to me as a kid. And when I retell the stories, I no longer relive the event. It just was - I've learned the lesson and moved on.

For example, say you were not allowed to do something when you were young that all the other kids could. When you think about that thirty-year-old plus illusion, it may bring up feelings of resentment toward your parents, grandma, or whoever you believed had "the power" over you back then. So, practice the NLP technique above a few times and see what happens. I'm willing to risk my M&M table setting collection that when you do this a few times - because once is rarely enough (notice I didn't say never?) that you'll begin to feel differently about it.

I used to be a counselor at a rehab home in southern California and I can say that the process of forgiveness was often a deal-breaker because not everyone is willing to forgive or be forgiven. That's exactly why it's important for you to look at these old illusions as ways to help you understand how you got to where you are today. Forgive yourself for allowing others to shadow your happiness with judgement, shame, or loathing. Claim your brilliance, and remember that the past is not the future, if you so choose. Train your habenula to reward you instead of keeping you stuck.

Reframe those memories in a way that helps you get the message and lesson to move on so you can keep looking forward to where your life is headed. We cannot live our lives in reverse. When we try to, basically, life sucks because it's a lot like trying to go forward while in reverse. Or it's like constantly looking over your shoulder, which can lead to some of the worst crashes.

What's cool about being human is that we're hardwired to survive. The downside is that looks a lot like homeostasis: the tendency toward a relatively stable equilibrium between interdependent elements, especially as maintained by physiological processes. This basically means change is bad.

That used to be "good" for us, because back in the day, if you left the tribe or cave, you could die. But today, not being able to change can encourage dis-ease. The stress of not being able to cope with change - jobs, technology, family dynamics, climate, and such - leads to a basket of dis-ease. Being flexible, open, and able to flow with change is challenging due to our "hard-wiring" but totally possible. How do you know it's possible? Because so many have already embraced this concept and are living proof. Can I give Millennials some props here?!

Your first step in affecting change in your life is to break the cycle with an action. Remember the baby steps? Could you get a "short" instead of a "venti"? Only order yourself a kid's meal at fast food joints? Or start taking a short walk immediately after dinner? Break the cycle of unhealthy with every small (Butterfly Effect) action you can think of. If you want a hundred and one tips, check out my first book, *Chocolate Cake for the Thighs.* What you did yesterday is not what you have to do today. You can make tomorrow a healthier place, first by choice, then by action. Choice without action is like a one-winged bird, and action without a healthy intention is the same.

Going forward, begin to forget how it "used to be" if "how it used to be" is how you got to be unhappy and unhealthy. Here's another fun assignment/opportunity. Take the time to think about the thoughts you have that are limiting. "We'll never get tickets. What if it rains? If we get lost? If we lose the game...blah, blah, blah." Then, ask the simple question that opposed those thoughts.

- Old: We'll never get tickets.
  New: What if we do or how can we?
- Old: What if it rains?

New: How can we plan for the weather? Or, just *expect* a glorious day!

- Old: What if we get lost?
  New: Um, how bout stop thinking that way – expectation follows thoughts
- Old: What if we lose?
  New: What if we win?

You get it. One of my favorite things about coaching people is, after listening patiently to all the reasons why they are where they are and don't have what they want, I ask "Well, what do you want?" I always get a kick out of the unique facial expressions that follows. It's almost like asking, "What's the best way to Mars?" And the best answer I could think of would be "up."

Keep your face to the sun, a song in your heart, and one foot in front of the other. And on occasion, when there is no sun, no song, and you stumble, then figure out why this happened, what your "role" in it was, and what's your next step is going to be. Or, just stay there in the dark, quiet and unmoving until you can't stand it anymore. The choice is yours. Famous motivational speaker Tony Robbins swears that everyone is either motivated by pleasure or pain. This is calorie-free food for thought.

I'd like to end this chapter with another super simple action you can do. Make your home a sanctuary. Begin by only bringing home food that supports your overall health and wellness. This way, when you want junk, there won't be any. Not only will you save money on your grocery bill, but you'll have less waste in your pantry and fridge. This will allow you to eat healthier because at first, you may not want carrot sticks, yogurt, or nuts. But after a while, you start to notice your skin and hair look more radiant, you're sleeping better, you don't feel "nappy" all the time, and your libido bounces back. After that, you'll be more inclined to make your home a sanctuary, motivated by pleasure.

True story: *You are a Badass* author and flag waver Jen Sincero loves to brag that she could get a parking space at the Vatican on Easter Sunday.

This is an awesome example of forgetting how it "used to be" or is only for others, and start believing in all you deserve – because you are so very deserving! I also have what I call great parking "Carma," and my good friend Caroline, calls her's rock-star parking. It is what it is, *and* it can also be yours.

Are you ready for the next step in your long-lasting happy and healthy life?

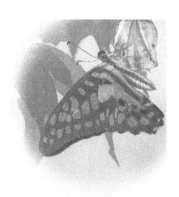

Chapter 11:

Now What?

While You're Alive,
There Can't Be a Final Step...

People like to quote Carnegie, Henry Ford, and Rockefeller, but back in the day, the real infamous motivational inspiration of the time was lesser known Florence Scovel Shinn*. While the gents were all about profit and success, Shinn *was* a prophet (vs profit). She understood that you had all the power you need in one single spot - your word. I highly recommend you read her work after you lay the groundwork for your action plan. Remember, you already know so much. However, she is my exception to the rule because perhaps you have never been privy to the knowledge, she "preaches". So please, just tuck this in your back pocket instead of just moving on to the next book as a distraction from action. Keep in mind that her work was published back in the early 1900s, so the language was a bit different. But the language and message still are very powerful. Never heard of her? Now you have! She was Christian based in her messages yet the stories she tells cross all faiths.

Now what? Go back to that first list of everything you know about how to be healthy and put a minus sign in front of everything you *know* that you are *not* doing/using, a check mark in front of all that you currently *are* doing, and a big star next to everything you honestly believe you can make a part of the way you live - forever.

Today, one of my favorite sayings is "Your word is your wand." It's the title of one of Florence Scovel Shinn's books, and when I first heard it, it resonated with me in a very powerful way. It's so important to remember how much power we have, and that ultimately, we make the majority of our own decisions even if we think we "have no choice." Begin speaking to yourself in a loving and kind way - always (yes, always!). And when you hear those little voices saying less than loving and support-ive things, tell them, "Stop it!" Or simply say, "Thanks for sharing, but I make the decisions and don't need you anymore."

There are lots of ways to do this. Get creative and come up with something powerful to tell those voices and let them know you are 100% in charge. Say what you want, not what you don't. Expect the best. Embrace it when it comes, and if it doesn't, learn the lesson and move on.

If you saw the movie *The Matrix*, you'll recall Samuel L. Jackson asks Keanu Reeves how far he's willing to go down the rabbit hole. Meaning, how much is he ready to learn. I'm telling you, "You've been living in the rabbit hole long enough!" It's time to come out in the sun and start putting all that knowledge to work. I know you think you have been doing that, but what's really been happening is, you simply keep going in and out of the hole, just a teeny bit in both directions, and very little has changed. You have not committed to a better life. And here's why...

Why motivation is like caffeine -
and what you can do about it...

Let's begin with a personal question, shall we? Are you a self-improvement junkie? Do you read the books, listen to podcasts, watch the TED talks, go to the seminars, *yet* after it's all said and done, you're basically the same person? Or, perhaps you have improved but still feel unfulfilled - like you are meant for something grander, more meaningful?

If the answer is "yes" then the following information can help you understand how to go from junkie to practitioner.

But, if the answer is "no" then you can relish in the fact that you can leap past that quagmire and just begin living your life on purpose, by design.

Now let's get started. Going from crash to flow is as easy as one-two-three.

First, it helps to understand that we are "wired" for security, and that knowing is enough. Knowing is not dangerous or life threatening, whereas, *doing* can lead to all sorts of unknown factors including failure, loss, financial ruin, and even death - or so we believe because that's what others or the statistics tell us. It's true that for thousands of years, if a person left the tribe to follow someone, it was *known* they never returned and were assumed dead. Yet we really did not *know*, it just made *sense*. On the other hand, perhaps they found greatness, a more loving tribe, or started something new. Have you ever wanted to leave your tribe/life behind and begin a quest for something more desirable?

Just take a moment right now and think about how much you *already* know about what you desire...better health, relationships, mindset, and such. If you're feeling extra motivated about understanding how to keep your motivation flowing, get a notebook and journal it. Getting it *out of your head and on paper* is the *first* step in making this happen. Then take that knowledge and make a Grand Plan for Success (your personal GPS) - you already know everything you need but keep reading. Once you have your GPS, reverse engineer it. That's when you go from ninety to, sixty, forty-five, then thirty, and finally *daily* actions to make this happen. Be realistic in your timeline. Some Grand Plans for Success take years - like becoming a chiropractor - where others can be accomplished much faster. And it's encouraged to have mini-Grand Plans (accomplishments) in your journey. This is really the Grand Plan!

How is this different from goals? It's unique in the fact that it's more of a plan for action. Generally, when people make goals, they look more like this: "I'm going to lose ten pounds this month." Goals are not always broken down and reverse engineered because that takes the romance out of them. Now wait! I'm a huge fan of romance but not in your GPS. You can for sure have lots of fun along the way, as long as you have a "way".

Along these same lines, the opposite is true for all your notes from seminars, workshops, and such. Set aside thirty minutes a day for ten straight days and find all those "gems" you documented and put the ones that still resonate with you *now* in one notebook so you can use them to help create and reverse engineer your GPS. Then - and this is very important - toss all those old files, journals, handouts, and notes. Clear some clutter and make room for your new experiences. Side note: if you have any self-help on cassette, VHS, or DVD, convert them to digital as part of your ten-day plan so you can access them easily across devices.

Next, get your Grand Plan for Success in your planner! Allow yourself some flexibility, but here is the non-negotiable part - get an accountability partner or coach. Your motivation will crash after those ten days like an energy drink in the wrong time zone if you fail to take this crucial support step! Make sure your partner understands what "accountability" means. You are not accountable if your partner allows excuses. Need help with this core step? Email me info@truespeak.us to git-er-duhn. One of the most powerful ways to stay in flow is to share your vision with like-minded people who can support you verses people who fear change and prefer to play small - happy with "good enough."

Finally, you will *stop* bringing in new information until you truly feel like you are "stuck" and seem to be experiencing trouble with your GPS. This is either an indication that you are ready to level up because it's time to learn what you are now ready to know. Or, it's time to re-evaluate your actions to see if any corrections are necessary because sometimes, we just don't know exactly how to get somewhere until we are physically – not mentally - on the journey. Knowledge is not power, applied knowledge is power. Begin *living* what you *already* know. Out of everything there is to "know" out there, it called to you for some reason, yet you have left it dormant, forgotten, or unapplied because of some unfounded personal fear. Or perhaps you gave it a shot so you could say "I tried that but...blah, blah, blah." Interesting how we will knowingly keep doing things that do not support our greater good - forever - yet we'll try something "good for us" just a few times before giving up so we can say we *tried*.

The only exception to this final step would be if you emotionally felt "called" to something via intuition or a gut feeling. You need to understand that while you keep seeking motivation from others (externally) and don't put the pedal to the metal for yourself, you will continue to live the motivational roller coaster and, the yo-yo of weight gain and loss.

Here is an example of a GPS and its process to achievement.

"I want to lose forty-five pounds this year and get off my hypertension and high cholesterol meds."

This kind of desire reminds me of when we wanted to get to the moon back in the day. We did not do it overnight. It was reverse engineered into baby steps.

Begin by getting your blood work done so you know what "distance" you must cover to get there. Make sure to ask your doctor what healthy numbers would look like for you and if there are options that can lead to getting off your meds.

Next, you'll set the daily intentions for eating healthier and doing the movement you love as well as restricting your screen time (across *all* devices). You know these are the best first steps. I'm just putting them here in case your brain does not want change and is freezing up on you. If you don't want to begin here, you're choosing to not change your habits to a healthy lifestyle. It's like saying, "I don't want to work. Just give me the money."

After that, you'll set monthly accomplishments to hit. Keep in mind, the first ten pounds are the easiest to lose.

After that, you must want it! Remember, you are creating a new paradigm for yourself. You are creating a life that supports your health and happiness - forever.

As you travel on this new adventure, there may be bumps, detours, or delays. Just know that you have the power to adapt and get back on course. Always encourage yourself like you would a child. This is new for you. Encouragement leads to lasting success, whereas chastising, blaming, and finger wagging lead to the destruction of your beautiful plan.

Every thirty days evaluate how it's going and decide if any adjustments need to be made to help get you exactly where you want to be. Pat yourself on the back often and yell out "Yay me!" when you do well. Watch out for rewarding yourself with "bad" food choices or a day off. You don't need a day off because this is just how you live now and forever. It may be challenging at first, but soon you'll see how it just becomes you.

Watch the inspirational movie *Heavenly Figures* starring Octavia Spencer and Kirsten Dunst to see what serious reverse engineering looks like.

Bonus: Understand that, in order for this to not be another motivational fix, you must take a moment right now - this very moment, no excuses - and close your eyes (after reading the instructions). Sit tall and begin breathing bigger, deeper, longer, and slower than normal. Take about three to five rounds of this deep inhale, expanding your lungs, belly, and ribcage, followed by a slow intentional exhalation that allows you to really let go. Then open your eyes and finish the exercise.

Notice how you feel and connect to that peace - without judgement about how you *think* you should feel. If you got a Grand Vision (Grand Visions are intuitive), jot it down. If not, do this again later in a more relaxed environment. And listen for your true voice, not the chatty ego. Be patient if it takes a few *tries*. Stay with it until you get from *trying* to *doing*. Then you can activate your GPS, the steps, the ten days, and accountability.

If for any reason or excuse you fall out of this process, start over with the breaths and get clear again on your Grand Plan for Success. The Vision may lead to some tweaking in your timeline. Allow your desire to keep you in flow – every day. Then adapt your action steps when necessary and work them. If you are not doing something every day (at least one action) that supports that Grand Vision, start over so you can see if you really desire this plan. If the answer is "yes," then tell whomever is subconsciously sabotaging you to "Stop it and get lost!" because everyone is either on board or off, without exception. Claim your power.

Review:

- Step one - Get the inspired Grand Plan/Vision with timeline.
- Step two - Get it in your planner and find an accountability partner/coach.
- Step three- Stop distracting yourself with more information and excuses.

Bonus: Slow down and relax with the breaths as often as possible (preferably daily).

Allow yourself to feel the flow of living your truth every day, without distraction. Breathe in the peace and joy of who you are and why you are here...and if you can't cold turkey the motivational stuff, then read this book over and over again until you are actually doing the assignments and living the lessons.

Another movie I recommend is *What the Bleep Do We Know*. Staring Marlee Matlin. It's an insightful and humorous look at all we don't know (or want to know), especially about our addictions, and food can be an addiction.

I'd like to end this chapter on a fun note. Did you know that all snowflakes look identical when they begin? Yup, but it's their own unique process of how they fall through the atmosphere that makes them one of a kind. Basically, no two snowflakes can have the same atmospheric experience. Just like us humans! We each have our own journey to claim as how we became the literal walking talking miracle that we are - beautiful.

True story: Back in the late eighties, I was hooked on self-improvement and was part of a "club" where I received one motivational cassette (I did say it was the 80's) a month. One month I received *Your Erroneous Zone* by Dr. Wayne Dyer. Well, I thought it was a bunch of hogwash and returned it - because I could. And I can't even remember what got instead. The point is, fast forward twenty years and I pick up the book - forgetting all about how I hated it before - next thing you know, I'm inspired by it, bought it for several people and still consider it one of my all-time favorites. Did the content change? Nope! I was just a different snowflake ready for the message.

As you can imagine, the time has come for you to make some R.E.A.L. decisions *and* put them into action....

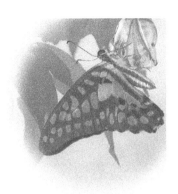

Conclusion:

NOT GOOD LUCK OR GOODBYE, BUT GOOD LIFE

You're Never on Your Own. Remember That.

You've made it this far because you love yourself and you are ready to get *real* about change. You now understand *why* things went down the way they did and *how* you can be large and in-charge instead of at the mercy of others and old thoughts/programming.

You have confidence because you see how you know so much and can make happy and healthy decisions every day - because you want to, not because someone else is telling you or guilting you.

You have a firm grasp of the E.M.P.A.T.H.Y. Way and how it can keep you moving forward. Because you have the notebook(s), made the lists, narrowed them into intentions and actions, and know your weaknesses. There is so much in here to accomplish that you promise yourself, you won't read another book, watch a TED Talk, or listen to one more podcast on the subject of weight loss or motivation until you work these processes and make at least three of them related to the way you live. This time you choose to make a difference instead of hiding behind all the lies and misdirection of your past. It's time to live the expression, "The buck stops here." with your new lifestyle of healthier food choices, movement, and happy thoughts.

"Good luck" would imply a kind of sarcastic tone. And even though I mean it sincerely, it still means you're mostly on your own, which you never are totally, unless you choose to be. You always have your higher power, True Source, and God light - you know that.

If you're ready to take your health back and to the next level, it's best done with a benevolent coach. Someone who understands your struggle but will no longer allow you to live in the past and blame others or circumstances. Someone who is more than a good listener. Someone who is trained in the art of calling you out by keeping you honest about your process and the steps *you* choose to get to where you desire and beyond (your personal GPS). There is hope for lasting success, you can feel it in your heart, and you know now is the time. You also know you're ready for a team now.

I suppose I'd be remiss if I didn't mention the third option - because inaction is also a choice you have the power over. You could choose to make this just another book in the long line of self-help, motivational, weight loss stuff you've been building an arsenal with. But I hope not.

Doing it alone has been challenging. It's time to enjoy the journey.

Are you inspired and ready to take actions that are either baby steps or leaps of faith? I sure hope so. If you find it difficult to stay in the happy-healthy zone, just remind yourself of how much time you have spent in the "unhealthy zone" and have a little patience for your shift. It will happen when you push through the resistance and redefine your homeostasis.

Here is a quick refresher: Homeostasis involves three parts:

1. the receptor - your thoughts
2. the control center - your emotions
3. the effector - your actions

Therefore, if you ever feel out of control, remember the saying for if you're on fire "Stop, Drop, and Roll" yourself back to your thoughts, or part one, so you can save yourself from getting burned again.

At a minimum, promise me you will commit to these three actions:

- Remember you are literally a walking, talking, breathing miracle
- Never go on a fad diet again or drink a diet soda
- Get an accountability partner

And finally, I can't say "It goes without saying" if I'm going to say it so here it goes...get that highlighter, a notebook for your GPS, a happiness journal, and read this book a few more times as you refine the assignments/opportunities down to real actions that show empathy for your body today. This ensures that you'll move from self-help junkie or sloth to superstar!

Then next year, when you visit your doctor and they complement you and ask what diet you went on, tell them "The Happiness Diet," because it's calorie free and lasts a lifetime!

I'd like to close with another true story because it's my favorite...I could never tell it as passionately as Becky Sampson. So here it is, in her words.

Never in a million years did I think I could break free from a lifetime of struggling with my weight.

Ever since I can remember, food has been my world. I thought about it, I ate it, and I used it as a way to comfort myself when I was happy, sad, angry, or excited. It was the one thing I felt I could "control" or, at least it felt that way. I stole money from my parents to buy candy, I hid wrappers in my dresser drawers, I snuck out to the local gas station to stash up and many times stuffed myself and had a hard time breathing. I was hoping that if I ate enough junk food, I would get so sick, I would never want it again. I was in a world of denial that kept me from seeing and truly connecting with others. It was a very lonely and painful world.

By age twelve, I was kneeling at my bedside pleading with God to take this obsession from me but thinking, 'I got myself into this problem, I'll have to get myself out of it.' Why would God care about my food anyway? It was then that I knew I was on my own and I couldn't dare ask for help. I internalized everything people said to me and became incredibly frightened by showing any weakness.

At age fifteen, I wanted the pain to end. I was convinced I was the cause of other's problems and a burden to those around me. I sat on my bedroom floor, holding my family picture, tearing little pieces of black electric tape and making a cross over my face all while reciting the words, "I want to die, I want to die, I want to die." I was hoping if I said it enough times, God would listen and take me. As a teenager, I wanted more than anything to fit into my family and among my friends and I wasn't feeling like anything I did was working.

A couple of hours went by, my heart was heavy, my eyes sore from the tears and my body absolutely exhausted. Feeling defeated, I finally fell asleep. I never told anyone of that night for fear of what they would think of me but instead I suffered for years in silence. My mother especially was very concerned about my weight and the things I was eating and would often threaten me with the comment, "If you don't eat better, you'll end up with diabetes." You would think that would inspire me as a teenager to turn my life around and start eating better, but no, when she'd hover over me with her comments about my food, it would make me want to eat even more.

In high school, I found solace when I ate, so I ate a lot in private and you know what they say, what you eat in private, shows in public. As I watched my friends go to prom, and make plans for their futures, as my self-esteem fell further and further down to where I never felt I would ever amount to anything important.

For years after that, I continued to struggle up and down and up and down the scales as I mustered up the motivation to lose weight. I tried it all, from diets to workout programs to personal trainers to training and running a marathon, all of which would work for a period of time but never gave me real relief from a lifetime of binging and overeating. It was more like white knuckling it until I didn't have an ounce of willpower left. Then, weighing in at my heaviest weight of two hundred and sixty-six pounds, I had no idea my life was about to change so drastically. I didn't see it coming, I didn't plan it out, I didn't put the date on the calendar saying, "I'll find the solution to all my problems today." It just happened.

Back in 2009, my sixty-eight-year-old, four foot eleven, Pilipino friend and I were walking around the mall getting our daily exercise when she turned to me and said, "I've eaten 4 cookies and need a detox." My first thought was, "Four cookies? That's nothing, more like two bags of cookies before I would even consider needing a detox." She then proceeded to beg me to come with her to a conference for food addicts in Las Vegas the following day. In a moment of spontaneous decision, I made the arrangements I needed - with her help - and before I knew it, we were on our way. After all, I was just going to support my friend in her time of need, so what the heck.

We arrived late and were filling out the registration information at the back of the room when I heard the speaker telling "my" story. I stopped what I was doing, and it was in that moment everything *changed. "Is this what I've struggled with my entire life? A food addiction? As speaker after speaker got up and told their story, I looked around the room and thought "Who are these crazy people and how do I get what they have?" which at the time, I didn't realize was recovery.*

I committed to the process and released one hundred-thirty pounds in fourteen months without any surgery, pills or exercise. That was over ten years ago. Although it hasn't been a perfect journey, I am maintaining my weight loss and am incredibly proud of the work I have done to get to this point.

And, my doctor recently gave me a clean bill of health.

We never know when an opportunity will come that gives us the very thing we have sought after our entire lives. I invite you, when you get inspired, take action, don't question and never look back unless you are looking back to see how far you have come. Namaste!

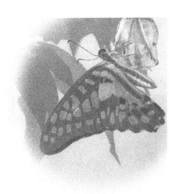

ACKNOWLEDGEMENTS

I t's true when they say, "It takes a village" (and a vineyard) to accomplish grand things in life.

The tribe that helped make this second book possible includes all the faithful ladies from the Oahu and Honolulu Clubs, for always being there for me, complimenting me, and showing up even in the rain.

And I'm blessed to have close family who love and appreciate me. Thank you, my dear loved ones for always encouraging me 100%. Especially when I want to dive into the deep end.

The foundation of this book was laid by my mentor and friend of nearly thirty years, Dr. Libby Adams, the founder of the International Academy of Self Knowledge (IASK) where I became a coach and certified in NLP and Transformational Meditation (TfM).

Huge props go out to Angela Lauria and my entire talented tribe at The Author Incubator for allowing me to focus on the message while they tended to the details of successful writing.

Mahalo to David Handcock, CEO and founder of Morgan James for believing in my message. I'm also so appreciative of my skilled publishing team: Jim Howard who helped make the vision clear for me, Amber Parrott who's creativity brought the book visually to life, and Gayle West who kept me on track and had answers to all my questions. Always. Thank you for making us "traditional readers" happy with a printed book!

And finally, yet most true to my heart, I'd like to acknowledge my two adult offspring Lexington Rose and Jaz Prime for giving me the endurance to see this through by constantly reminding me how proud they are of their Momma.

Looking forward to the audio book coming this year as well as all the amazing butterfly and ripple effects that have been put into play. Oh, and of course, book number three! Aloha to all.

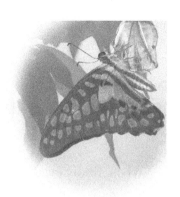

THANK YOU

Applause and high-fives all around! I so appreciate you and your commitment to honor yourself and your body going forward in life. You now have an arsenal of tools to use on your adventure to become happier and healthier.

Remember, it's important to use those tools daily. Never again will you wonder why something happened to you or use blame as a crutch to stay stuck. Why use the heel of a shoe when you have a hammer, or your thumbnail when you have a screwdriver to get the job done right? The list of things you've gleaned from this book are for your adaptation – thank you. This is my wish for you dear reader. It's now, onward and upward, face to the sun with a smile on your face and a song in your heart – forever.

Your Gifts

When you're ready for a coach, reach out to me for a *complimentary* strategy session on your GPS at **info@ Truespeak.us**

Also, because you made it to the final words, I'm offering you the additional gifts of the e-book *The Positive Purpose of Negative Emotions*, plus the pdf of *Why Motivation is like caffeine – and what you can do about it*. Simply email me at info@Truespeak.us and put "I gotta have it!" in the subject box.

And, of course, if you have a group you know would benefit from my message, please reach out because I'd love to come share it with you – no matter where you may be on the planet. I LOVE to travel!

I honor your journey and am already so very proud of you.

Your friend in health and happiness,

Ell

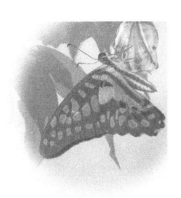

About the Author

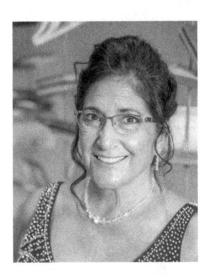

E ll Graniel has a passion for motivation that began over thirty-five years ago when she became a certified group fitness instructor, manager, and key-note speaker for such influential companies as 24-Hour Fitness and Beach Body's Chalene Johnson.

In 1996 she began training with the International Academy of Self-Knowledge (IASK) where she earned her certification as a coach, NLP, and Transformational Meditation™ (TfM) Facilitator.

Shortly after that, Ell earned her B.A. degree in Communication and started Truespeak™, her unique business specializing in how to get what you want just by asking.

The success of her coaching comes from the blend of the relationship between Neuro-Linguistic Programming (NLP), the different languages of learning styles, and quantum physics that has been gleaned from decades of research and documentation.

Her motto is, "Say what you want. The truth is in you."

She currently resides in Honolulu, Hawaii where she enjoys sunsets on the beach, reading, writing, and her infamous disco ball collection.

Her first book Chocolate Cake for the Thighs – the anti-diet book for women was published in 2006 and she has also penned articles for several publications.

Ell is also a keynote speaker, podcast guest, blogger, and presenter on topics such as motivation, communication skills, healthy living, and NLP.

She may be reached at:

Website: https://www.truespeak.us/

Page: EllGraniel.com

Email: info@truespeak.us

And followed on:

Facebook: https://www.facebook.com/2truespeak/

IG: 4Truespeak
YouTube: Ell Graniel
Twitter: Truespeak@EllGraniel

Truespeak™ is the language the "observer" speaks in your mind and is the one directly connected to your higher power. When you learn how to meditate, you strengthen that connection. Guided meditation is the first step toward that accomplishment. Truespeak™ also teaches you how to connect with your higher power to resolve conflict, turmoil, and unresolved issues in your thoughts and actions.

Mind Body Language (MBL) is the classroom style learning about how the voices in your head control your actions and attitudes and how to take back that control and put peace in your corner again.

Educational institutions, organizations, and corporations are just a few of the types of clients for which she trains and presents the MBL theories. Some of her diverse clientele includes University of Hawaii, Hawaii Health at Work Alliance, Houghton-Mifflin, Beachbody, BNI, and IDEA Health & Fitness association.

Her forte is keynote speaking, as her approach is direct, and her humor and insight are refreshing and enlightening.

In 1989, Ell created Image-makers & Seminars, a professional image consulting and training company. In 1996 she morphed that company and founded Truespeak™. Ell has her B.S. in Business Communication, is certified in Transformational Meditation™ (TfM), holds multiple fitness certifications, and has training in Neuro-Linguistic Programming, Myers-Briggs Type Indicator, and The Enneagram Type Indicator.

To date, she has produced, starred in, and hosted a variety of television programs. Her insights have been quoted in newspapers, and magazines such as Family Fun, and IDEA Fitness Journal. And her book Chocolate Cake for the Thighs – the anti-diet book for women is still available on Amazon.

Truespeak™ is the language in which one expresses what they want vs. what they don't. Truespeak™ would say, "remember your lunch," instead of, "don't forget your lunch." Or, "How can I improve my situation?" instead of, "Why does this always happen to me?" When you ask better questions, you get better answers.

Since our words are the direct manifestation of our thoughts, wouldn't it be more valuable to think and state what you want in life rather than what you don't? Remember, it's your mind, your life, and you're in charge. You have the power.

Learn how your language can move you in a more powerful & successful direction. Her training teaches you how the mind processes information and how the use of Truespeak™ can realize your goals on many levels. Learn to identify your limiting internal and external language and how to replace it with Truespeak™. Good things come to those who ask.

Say what you want. The truth is in you.

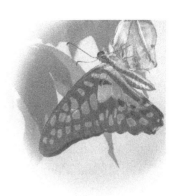

RECOMMENDED & STARRED REFERENCES *

Books:

- Your Erroneous Zones by Dr. Wayne Dyer (or any and all of his books)
- The Complete Writings of Florence Scovel Shinn
- Spontaneous Happiness by Dr. Andrew Weil (or any and all of his books)
- Jurassic Park by Michael Crichton
- Chocolate Cake for the Thighs by L Kae Graniel
- You Are a Badass by Jen Sincero

Movies:

- Groundhog Day
- What the Bleep Do We Know

- Hidden Figures
- Hector and the Pursuit of Happiness

Facts to Google:
- Zig Ziglar
- Muscle Memory
- Cortisol
- Visceral Fat
- NLP
- Morph Types
- The Habenula
- Hydrostatic Body Fat Testing
- History of the Food Guide Pyramid

Apps:
- Fooducate (for reading and defining food ingredients on labels, *not* counting calories)